NATUROPATHIC PHYSIOTHERAPY

C. P. Negri, OMD, ND

Infinity Health Care Books

NATUROPATHIC PHYSIOTHERAPY
By C. P. Negri, OMD, ND

Printed in the United States of America.

ISBN: 978-1-7372929-5-1
Care has been taken to confirm the accuracy of the information presented in this work. While the subject matter of this book contains generally accepted practices in several licensed healthcare professions, many are not accepted in the practice of mainstream medicine and do not represent the consensus of medical opinion at this time. The reader should be aware of this and the author and publisher are not responsible for errors or omissions, or for the consequences from the application of the information in this book and make no warranty, express or implied, with respect to its contents. It is the responsibility of each provider to ascertain the current status of, and possible complications from, any and all procedures that are given or recommended.

also by C. P. NEGRI:

Green Medicine
Naturopathic Treatment of Blood Pressure
Naturopathic Treatment of Emotional Illness
A Century of Naturopathy
Why Natural Therapies Work (and How to Make Them Work Better)
Naturopathic Joint Mobilization
The Negri Manual of Natural Medicine, Vol. I and Vol.II

DEDICATION

To **J. Murl Johnston, MD,**
Homeopath and master of physical medicine,
This volume is respectfully dedicated

CONTENTS

Foreword

As a physical therapist, I entered this profession with a deep desire to help people improve mobility, live stronger, and truly heal. From the start, I loved being part of someone's recovery - watching them go from pain and limitation to strength and confidence. But over the years, something started to change. We shifted from individualized, hands-on care to something that feels more like an assembly line.

Too often, patients are cycled in and out, checked off a list, and sent home with a standard exercise packet. A once personal and rewarding process has become burdened by time constraints, productivity metrics, and overwhelming documentation demands. I often found myself frustrated, knowing that many patients needed more than what the system allowed me to give.

Then something unexpected happened. I was introduced to Naturopathy.

Until that moment, I'll be honest, I didn't even know what a naturopathic doctor was. It was never mentioned in physical therapy school. We were never taught that there were other providers using many of the same modalities; diathermy, iontophoresis, hydrotherapy, and other tools designed to reduce inflammation and promote healing.

Learning about Naturopathy opened my eyes to a completely different way of thinking about health. It reminded me that healing isn't just physical - it's whole-body, inside and out.

Alicia Fancher, MPT

Preface

Naturopathy, as envisioned by its founder, was characterized by "pathological monism, therapeutic universalism". In other words, there was fundamentally one cause of disease, but *every* means of dealing with it—as long as it was natural—was the naturopathic doctor's legacy.

In 46 years of practice, there are few therapies I have not used, at least occasionally. Most patients, though, have wanted me to *prescribe*, because that is what the dominant medical profession does, and what the pharmaceutical industry tells them they want. Regardless, I have insisted in most cases on coupling the use of natural medicines with the most appropriate type of physiotherapy that fits the case; whether it be hydrotherapy, spinal mobilization, acupuncture, infrared or ultraviolet light, or corrective exercises.

Recently, a Physical Therapy authority listed the "twenty-three most indispensable tools for PT". I was taken aback when I saw the list and the weight given to them. They were:

1. Treadmill	12. Adjustable Tables
2. Stationary Bicycle	13. Cuff Weights
3. Resistance Bands	15. Balance Discs
4. Dumbbells	16. Pulley Systems
5. Exercise Balls	17. Therapeutic Putty
6. Balance Boards	18. Ankle and Wrist Weights
7. Foam Rollers	19. **Ultrasound Machines**
8. Therabands	20. **Electrical Stimulation Devices**
9. Pedal Exercisers	21. Vibration Plates
10. Hand Grippers	22. **Heat Packs**
11. Parallel Bars	23. **Nebulizer Equipment**

As one can clearly see from this list, the modern Physical Therapist has a role more like an exercise physiologist or an athletic trainer than a health care provider. After the exhaustive list of motor fitness aids, only four of the 23 are modalities that are covered in this book—and they are at the bottom of the list!

In Chapter One, I include a short history of the use of physiotherapy in the naturopathic and other fields, and its transformation into the allied medical profession now known as Physical Therapy. Because the term *physiotherapy* ceased to be used in mainstream healthcare, there has always been some confusion when naturopathic doctors like myself refer to it (indeed, I once was investigated by the State Board of Physical Therapy for encroaching on their turf).

Having had cordial relations with many physical therapists over the years and having had some as students, I felt I was fairly familiar with the practice. Unknown to me, over the years Physical Therapy appears to have largely discarded much of *physiotherapy* in its original form, in favor of a focus on rehabilitation and occupational therapy.

It is that original form of physiotherapy that naturopathic doctors (NDs) preserve. It is up to you now, to guard them from extinction.

C.P. Negri, OMD, ND
2025

1

Historical Use of Physiotherapy in Naturopathy

> **physiotherapy**
>
> /fĭz"ē-ō-thĕr'ə-pē/
>
> **noun**
>   1.   therapy that uses physical agents: exercise and massage and other modalities

In the early years of the 20th Century, when mainstream medicine was moving rapidly away from forms of treatment that did not involve the new synthetic drugs, trouble was brewing. There were three major challengers to the conventional medical profession and all of them considered themselves "drugless"—naturopaths, osteopaths, and chiropractors.   Osteopaths and chiropractors believed in healing by way of the musculoskeletal system and applied the hands to correct structural flaws. Naturopaths did likewise; but included in their armamentarium was a vast array of other modalities they did not hesitate to use in their philosophy of "therapeutic universalism".

Osteopaths began to use physiotherapy modalities to augment their manual treatment (eventually moving on to pharmaceutical drugs and minimizing the importance of manipulation). Some chiropractors incorporated physiotherapy into their practices and became ostracized by the fountainhead of Chiropractic, which decreed "By hand alone!"   Thus the profession became split into the orthodox "straights" and the "mixers".

But the naturopaths possessed something unique: Their right to use these modalities was enshrined in congressional law. Naturopathy was defined in 1931 as

> ...the diagnosis and practice of physiological and material sciences of healing, encompassing a wide range of natural therapies such as mechanotherapy, articular manipulation, corrective orthopedic gymnastics, neurotherapy, psychotherapy, hydrotherapy, mineral baths, electrotherapy, thermotherapy, phototherapy, chromotherapy, vibrotherapy, thalmotherapy, and dietetics.

Where, then, did Physical Therapy come from?

Naturopaths, osteopaths and chiropractors had gained favor with the public with their use of physical remedies, rather than chemical ones. Conventional medicine, while fighting these groups legislatively, increasingly prevented them from practicing, also used propaganda to steer people away from the "dangerous and unscientific" practices they offered. It was not completely successful. And because the American Medical Association noticed that the public was spending a lot of money for these therapies anyway, they decided that they weren't dangerous and unscientific at all—if a medical doctor performed them.

I learned this history from someone who was there at its inception. After graduation, I was fortunate to undertake preceptorships with several doctors who used a lot of physiotherapy. One had started his medical practice in 1928. He was in the vanguard of medical doctors who used these modalities and organized them into what they called "Physical Medicine". Dr. Murl Johnston detailed to me the conferences he attended that created the specialty that would come to be called *Physiatry*. However, physiatrists, or specialists in Physical Medicine, did not propagate as they had planned, because it was generally obvious that one would have a far more lucrative practice writing prescriptions than by applying time-consuming therapies like heat or electrotherapy.

Thus was birthed the allied health care profession of Physical Therapy. The medical doctor did not have to deliver the treatments; he simply had to order them done.

Bear in mind that there were multiple factors contributing to this change. One was that the osteopaths were being taken into the mainstream medical community as they abandoned the "drugless" mantle. Another was the dwindling number of naturopathic schools and the loss of licensure in many states that limited the ND's competition with the MD. Still another was the growing prevalence of health insurance paying for orthodox care. When formerly there had been no insurance footing the bill, people flocked to the low-cost and less invasive drugless doctor.

And finally, there was the gradual expansion of education required for every type of healthcare provider. Medical doctors were eventually required to have four years of medical school, plus internship, plus residency, adding up to eleven years of training (and expense), essentially eliminating the possibility of private practice after graduation for most. The modern doctor must work in the system that created him, and the hospital or conglomerate that holds his contract provides the ancillary services like Physical Therapy.

By contrast, my family doctor when I was a child graduated from a two-year program. MDs from both two- year and four-year schools were licensed when I was growing up.

As the complexity has increased, so has the number of support staff; there are medical assistants, outranked by physician assistants, and the nurse who once worked at the elbow of the doctor now has varying degrees of education (LPN, RN, LVN, ADN, BSN, MSN), and now even a Doctor of Nursing Practice. And she now has her very own Certified Nursing Assistant.

So it should puzzle no one how the physical therapist, once a lower-echelon provider, now has such lengthy and expensive schooling. The field has been so transformed that it is difficult to get into a Physical Therapy degree program today.

Where does that leave the Doctor of Naturopathy? While some naturopathic colleges have boosted their educational requirements and insisted on a more mainstream medical curriculum, most of those graduates—ironically—use little physiotherapy, preferring the prescription pad like the osteopaths before them. Traditional naturopathic colleges have resisted increasing the length, complexity, and cost of schooling in favor of concentrating on good training in simple therapies. What must be emphasized is that light, water, heat, pressure, and all the elements of physiotherapy contained in this book *work exactly the same as they did a hundred years ago,* and there is no reason for it to take a decade of learning in order to implement them. There is also no reason that a patient in need should have to go to a conventional medical facility to receive physiotherapy simply because the conventional group has popularized the term "Physical Therapy".

Naturopaths need to assertively regain their place in the delivery of these natural procedures that have become so well known in the age of sports medicine. Latter-day schools have been at a disadvantage because of so few qualified instructors, and many of the exclusively naturopathic textbooks have been out of print for years. This book is an attempt to begin turning that ship around.

Advice to the reader: Some of the methods here you will have had experience with; others, minimal or none. You should skim the book (as most will) and note the modality that most interests you. Read that section. Think about it for a time. Gather the materials for performing it and try it on yourself. If the results are positive, try another. With time and experience, you can add tools to your practice that greatly expand your ability to help people. That is what it *should be* all about.

An Act of Congress
Passed February 7, 1931

THE FOLLOWING DEFINITION OF NATUROPATHY was passed by the United States Congress on February 7, 1931, without a dissenting vote. There was very great opposition by 35 medical doctors present, by the Board of Commissioners of the Healing Act (allopathic), and by special representatives and attorneys of the American Medical Association and other allopathic forces.

"Section 2. It is further enacted that 'NATUROPATHY,' as used in the aforesaid Act, approved February 27, 1929, hereafter shall comprehend, embrace, and be composed of the following acts, practices, and usages, ---

"DIAGNOSIS and PRACTICE of physiological and material sciences of healing as follows, ---

"The physiological and mechanical sciences such as mechanotherapy, articular manipulation, corrective orthopedic gymnastics, neurotherapy, PSYCHOTHERAPY, hydrotherapy, and MINERAL BATHS, electrotherapy, thermotherapy, phototherapy, chromotherapy, vibrotherapy, thalmotherapy, and DIETETICS WHICH SHALL INCLUDE THE USE OF FOODS OF SUCH BIOCHEMICAL TISSUE-BUILDING PRODUCTS AND CELL SALTS AS ARE FOUND IN THE NORMAL BODY; and the use of vegetal oils and dehydrated and pulverized fruits, flowers, seeds, barks, herbs, roots, and vegetables uncompounded and in their natural state.

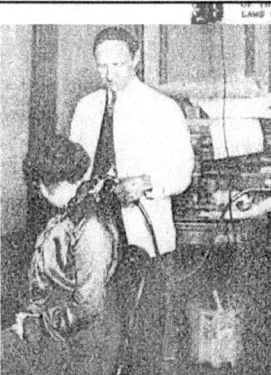

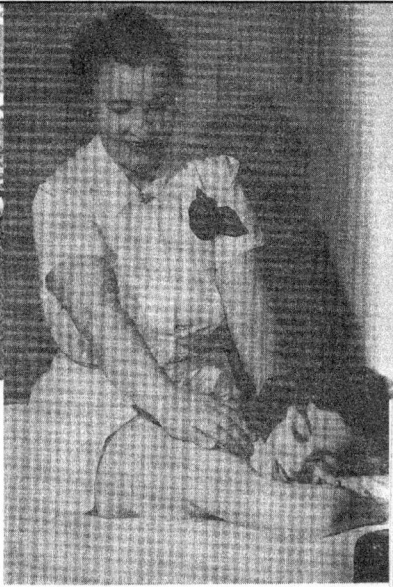

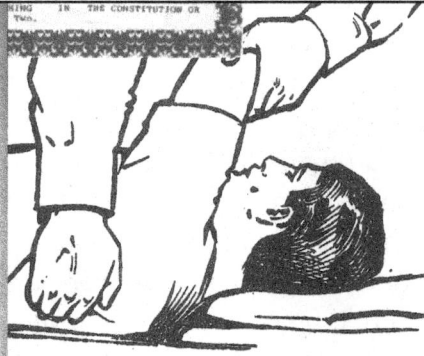

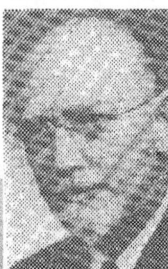

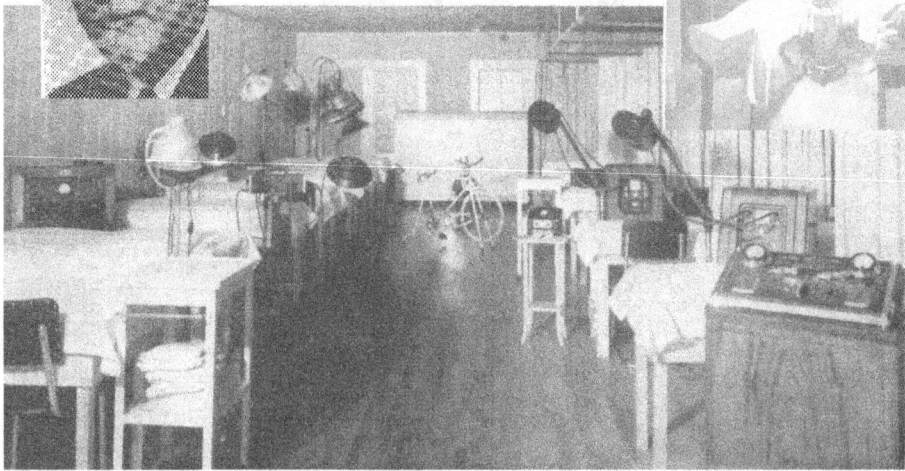

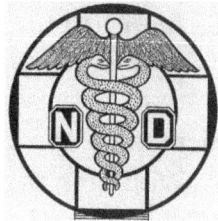

"Passed the House of Representatives February 7, 1931. Attest: Wm. Tyler Page, Clerk."

"Section 2. It is further enacted that 'NATUROPATHY,' as used in the aforesaid Act, approved February 27, 1929, hereafter shall comprehend, embrace, and be composed of the following acts, practices, and usages, ---

"DIAGNOSIS and PRACTICE of physiological and material sciences of healing as follows, ---

"The physiological and mechanical sciences such as mechanotherapy, articular manipulation, corrective orthopedic gymnastics, neurotherapy, PSYCHOTHERAPY, hydrotherapy, and MINERAL BATHS, electrotherapy, thermotherapy, phototherapy, chromotherapy, vibrotherapy, thalmotherapy, and DIETETICS WHICH SHALL INCLUDE THE USE OF FOODS OF SUCH BIOCHEMICAL TISSUE-BUILDING PRODUCTS AND CELL SALTS AS ARE FOUND IN THE NORMAL BODY; and the use of vegetal oils and dehydrated and pulverized fruits, flowers, seeds, barks, herbs, roots, and vegetables uncompounded and in their natural state.

4

2

THERMOTHERAPY: HEAT

OVERVIEW

Thermotherapy accelerates tissue healing by increasing the amount of oxygen that the target locations receive. The increase in oxygen enables tissues to increase the catabolic rate of destructive enzymes (e.g., collagenase), thus lessening their impact. Overall, these effects accelerate healing, improve blood circulation, and provide pain relief to patients. From hot cloths and hot water bottles to heating pads and infrared radiation, naturopaths use various tools to provide thermotherapy. There are three categories of heat used:

- Conductive—heat applied in contact with the body;
- Convective—heat from a source not in contact;
- Conversive— energy converted into heat in the tissues from a device (covered in the sections on diathermy and ultrasound)

CONDUCTIVE HEAT: HOT PACKS

DESCRIPTION

The usual type of conductive heat used by a typical naturopath is the hot pack. The commercial hot pack delivers moist heat to the patient's body. They are typically made of canvas and filled with a substance such as silica gel that retains the heat. It is warmed in a hydrocollator (a heated tank of water set to around 170°F). The hot pack can retain heat for about 30 minutes. Alternatively, stacked towels that have been soaked in hot water can be used without the need for a manufactured hot pack.

EQUIPMENT NEEDED

- Hydrocollator tank (or a container with a *sous vide* heating unit to heat the water)
- Hot packs in a variety of sizes (or thick Terry cloth towels hung on a rack in the water)
- A supply of Terry cloth towels, bath size

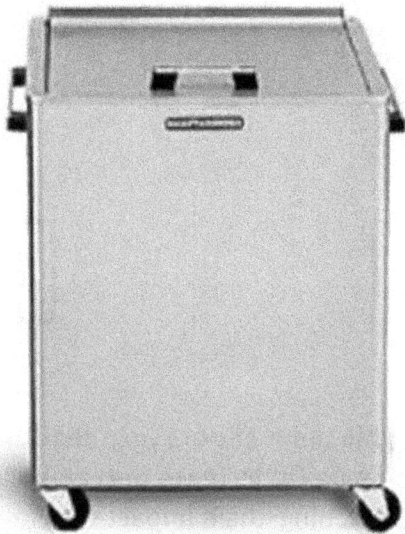
Chattanooga brand
Hydrocollator

EFFECTS AND PURPOSE
•Perspiration (and thus local detoxification) is induced.
•Local metabolism is increased.
•Local vasodilation is achieved.
•Muscle relaxation is induced.
•Sensory nerves are sedated, making subsequent therapies better tolerated.
•The preheating makes for a better response to subsequent electrotherapy.

INDICATIONS FOR USE
• Subacute or chronic inflammation
• Aid in systemic detoxification
• Aid to athletic recovery

CONTRAINDICATIONS
• Open wounds.
• Acute inflammation may be aggravated by heat therapy.
• Tissues with damage from X-ray treatment should not be heated.
• Bleeding within the myofascial tissues from recent trauma may be prolonged.
• Patients with peripheral vascular disease may not be able to handle the increased metabolic demands of heated body tissues.
• Anyone with impaired sensitivity.

PRECAUTIONS
• The elderly and young children (under four years of age) do not have reliable thermoregulatory systems and can develop fever as a result, which may be alarming if the healing power of hyperthermia is not explained.
• Confused patients who are unreliable judges of heat perception should only be treated every cautiously, if at all.
• Edematous patients may be aggravated if given too intense heating.

ADVANTAGES
• Low-tech, affordable equipment.
• Therapeutic for many conditions a naturopath would treat.
• Can treat multiple patients at a time.
• Renders manual therapy or electrotherapy even more effective.

DISADVANTAGES

- Plumbing (although simple) required.
- Towel service needed if one does not self-launder the towels.

INSTRUCTIONS

1. Always instruct the patient about the procedure and what to expect.
2. Have patient remove all clothing and jewelry from the area being treated.
3. Inspect skin in the area to be treated.
4. Position, patient comfortably and modestly. Cover the area under treatment with a clean towel.
5. Remove hot pack from water using the tabs and place on two Terry cloth towels, folded lengthwise and arranged as seen in the illustration. One can also use a commercially made terrycloth cover. These are readily available.

Hot pack

6. Fold the towels, making 6 to 8 layers of toweling covering the hot pack. Ensure that the tabs are covered by the toweling. If using a commercial cover, cover that with a clean towel.
7. Place pack on the area to be treated. Emphasize to the patient that the heat should be a comfortable level but not as hot as can be tolerated.
8. Cover the entire region with a sheet or additional towing.
9. Monitor the patient and add or remove toweling as needed for comfort. One should have a call button to alert the naturopath if he or she is out of the room. The practitioner should always be nearby to make any necessary changes and to periodically check the skin during the treatment.
10. Duration of treatment is 15 to 30 minutes, although if used to prep the body for other therapies, it is typically only applied for 10 to 15 minutes.
11. At the end of the session, remove the pack and dry the patient, checking the condition of the skin and the vascular response. Allow patient to rest while you return the hot pack to the heating unit.
12. Removing the toweling and depositing it in a hamper, return the hot pack to the heating unit and allow at least 30 minutes of reheating before using it again.

FREQUENCY OF TREATMENT

Hot packs may be given daily or even multiple times a day in subacute conditions. Always reduce the frequency of sessions as the patient improves.

REFERENCES

- Baruch, S., *An Epitome of Hydrotherapy*, W.B. Saunders Co., 1920
- Boyle, W., and Saine, A., *Lectures in Naturopathic Hydrotherapy*, Buckeye Naturopathic Press 1988
- Kellogg, J.H., *Rational Hydrotherapy*, F.A. Davis Co., 1903
- Kovacs, R., *A Manual of Physical Therapy*, Lea & Febiger, 3rd Edition 1946
- Krusen, F., *Physical Medicine*, 1941 W.B. Saunders Co.

THERMOTHERAPY: HEAT

T

CONVECTIVE or RADIANT HEAT

DESCRIPTION
Radiant heat and light from incandescent sources were common in naturopathic physiotherapy of years past; many devices were used, such as lamps with high wattage bulbs (illustrated at right) and whole cabinets filled with such filaments where the entire body could be bathed in light and heat (covered elsewhere in **Electric Light Bath**).

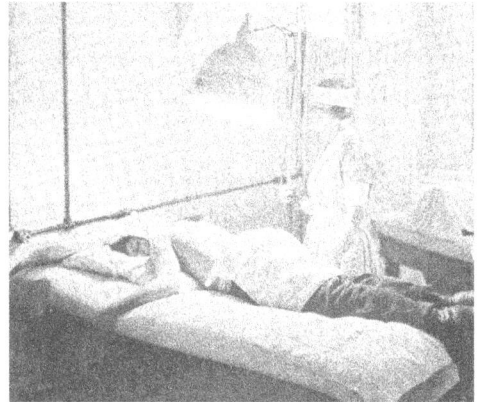

As physiotherapy progressed, use came to be made of other frequencies of light outside the visible spectrum that also had a heating effect, such as **Infrared**, also covered in a later chapter on **Phototherapy** (the technical information on infrared in this section is duplicated in the chapter solely on that modality).

Convective heat operates on a simple physical principle. It activates vasomotor reflexes that direct a greater volume of blood to be rushed to the part treated, simultaneously stimulating the expelling of as much of the excess heat as possible in an instinctive defense against tissue damage. The result is the reflex action can also take an action on adjacent and even distant parts of the body. Therefore, a more systemic response of increased blood flow and excretion of waste products in the tissues is created.

It is important to note that increasing the degree of heat applied will not cause a deeper penetration and affect underlying tissues, for the very reason explained above.

EQUIPMENT NEEDED
A radiant heat lamp, either luminous or non-luminous. Luminous bulbs are usually tungsten filament bulbs and produce mainly short wave (near) infrared waves. Non-luminous lamps are typically a carborundum core with a reflector, and produce mainly long wave (far) infrared waves.

9

Carbon arc lamps were one type of radiant heat used in Naturopathy in times past. This type of equipment was superseded over time and replaced by infrared lamps, and then the carbon arc lamps ceased being manufactured. They are mentioned for completeness.

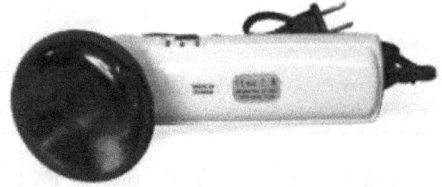

Infralux, a small hand-held device is easy to use and affordable.

EFFECTS AND PURPOSE

Long wave (far) infrared is absorbed in the stratum corneum of the epidermis, only 1-2 mm. Yet, they are known to reduce pain, accelerate skin healing, lower blood pressure, increase peripheral circulation, benefit chronic kidney disease, and modulate autoimmune responses. Their use in full-body saunas is well known today. They are in the frequency range of 2000 to 3,000 nanometers.

Short wave (near) infrared penetrates deeply, 5-10 mm, affecting vascular beds in the dermis and nerve endings. They affect arterial and venous circulation and they stimulate more perspiration than long wave infrared. They stimulate energy production in the mitochondria. They are in the frequency range of 780 to 3,000 nanometers.

INDICATIONS FOR USE
• Subacute or chronic inflammation
• Arthritis and other rheumatic conditions
• Neuritis, boils and carbuncles
• Aid in systemic detoxification
• Aid to athletic recovery
• Aid to peripheral circulation

CONTRAINDICATIONS
• Open wounds
• Dermatitis
• Swelling or bruising at site
• Multiple sclerosis patients
• Diabetic patients
• Patients with deep vein thrombosis (DVTs)
• Patients with other vascular diseases

PRECAUTIONS
• Patients with neurosensory problems cannot judge the level of heat, requiring careful monitoring of such patients. The same goes for patients with confusion.

- Existing edema can be aggravated by radiant heat. Mild intensity should be used, along with elevation.

ADVANTAGES
- No contact is made with the device, so no tenderness or balking at touch.
- The non-contact eliminates the contamination of wounds.
- The part treated can be continually monitored.

DISADVANTAGES
- Radiant heat cannot be used if the patient cannot be positioned properly to expose the target area.
- A small target area is difficult to irradiate due to the spread of the waves from the device to the body (although this can be remedied by a shroud made of cardboard with a hole the appropriate size cut into it) .

INSTRUCTIONS
1. Always check equipment first.
2. Non-luminous lamps should be turned on 5-10 minutes before application.
3. Explain the procedure to the patient. Have patient remove all jewelry and clothing from the area to be treated.
4. Drape the patient for modesty, but expose the area to be treated. Position the patient so that the target area for treatment is accessible.
5. Check patient's ability to sense heat and inspect skin for lesions that may preclude treatment.
6. Position the lamp in such way that a majority of the waves will hit the body at a right angle (perpendicular).
7. Measure the distance from the filament to the skin and record it in your notes.
8. Tell the patient that a comfortable warmth is the goal and not the limit that the patient can stand. Emphasize that patient should not move closer to the lamp or touch it. If unable to have constant monitoring, give patient a bell or other alarm to summon help if uncomfortable.
9. Treat for 15-20 minutes; a chronic condition needs 20-30 minutes.
10. Turn off and remove lamp. Dry the patient's skin and cover. Allow patient to rest for a few minutes before rising.

Note: The patient may adapt to the heat level after a time and request a higher intensity. *Moving the lamp closer risks burning the patient* because of the inability to judge it accurately.

Remember that the source-to-skin distance is what determines the amount of heat.

A non-luminous lamp (carborundum core) producing far infrared with a 750 to 1000 watt output should be placed 36 inches away, measured from skin to the filament, raising or lowering later as needed.

A luminous lamp of 1000 watts should be placed at 30 inches to start. Smaller bulbs (500-600 watts) can be placed at 24 inches and all can be raised or lowered as needed.

FREQUENCY OF TREATMENT

Daily, or even twice daily in subacute conditions. Chronic conditions should be treated once or twice a week.

REFERENCES

- Lehmann, et.al., Therapeutic Heat and Cold; Ed.3, 1982 Williams & Wilkins
- Kovacs, R., Light Therapy; 1950 Charles C. Thomas
- Johnson, A.C., Principles and Practice of Drugless Therapeutics; 3rd Ed., Chiropractic Educational Extension Bureau 1946
- Kellogg, J.H., Light Therapeutics; 1927 Modern medicine Pub. Co.

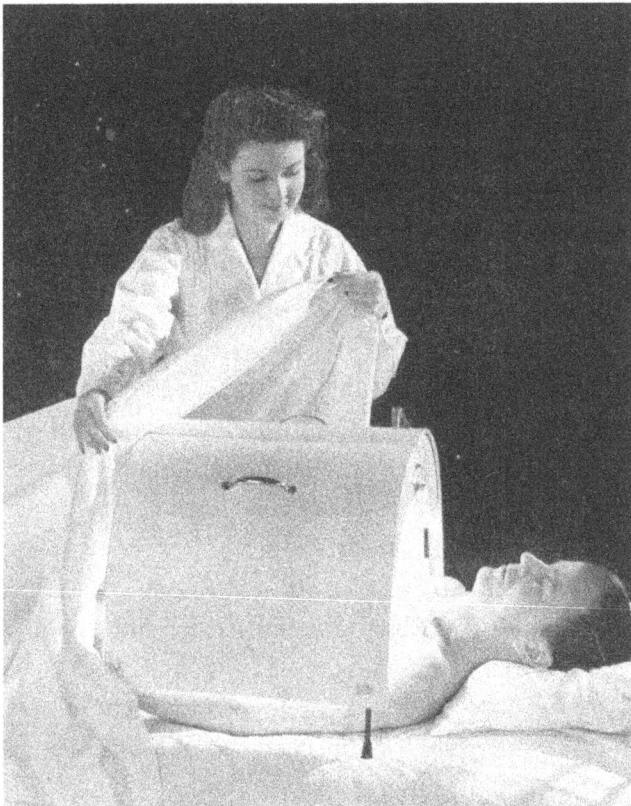

The once common "cradle baker" heat lamp

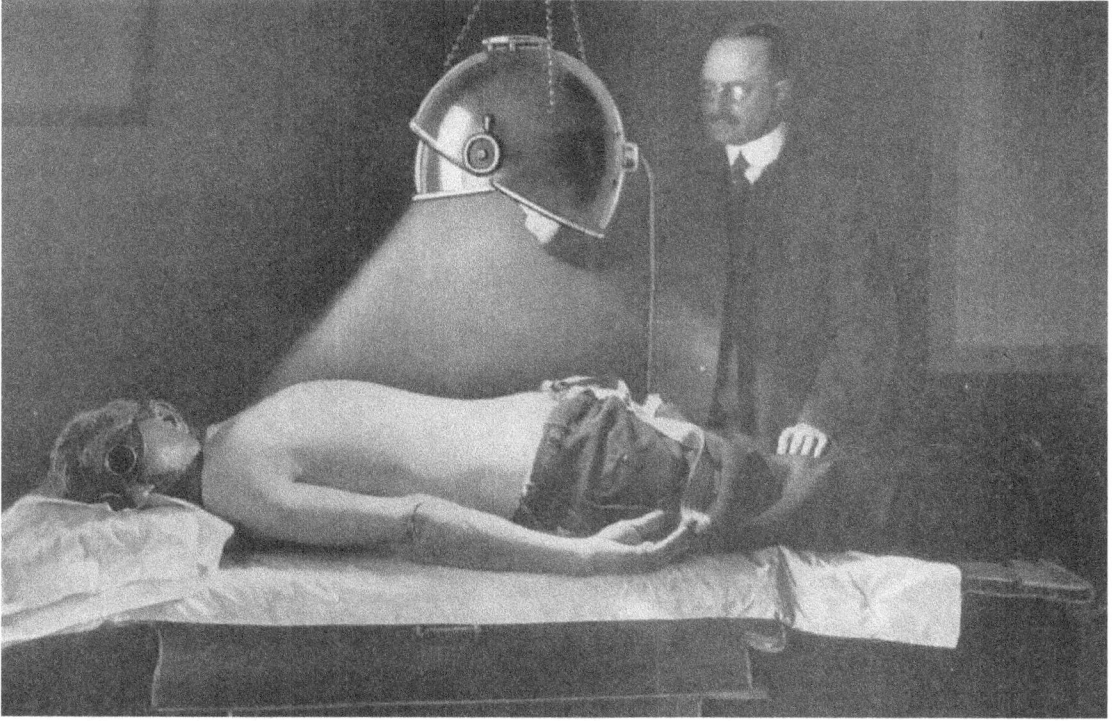

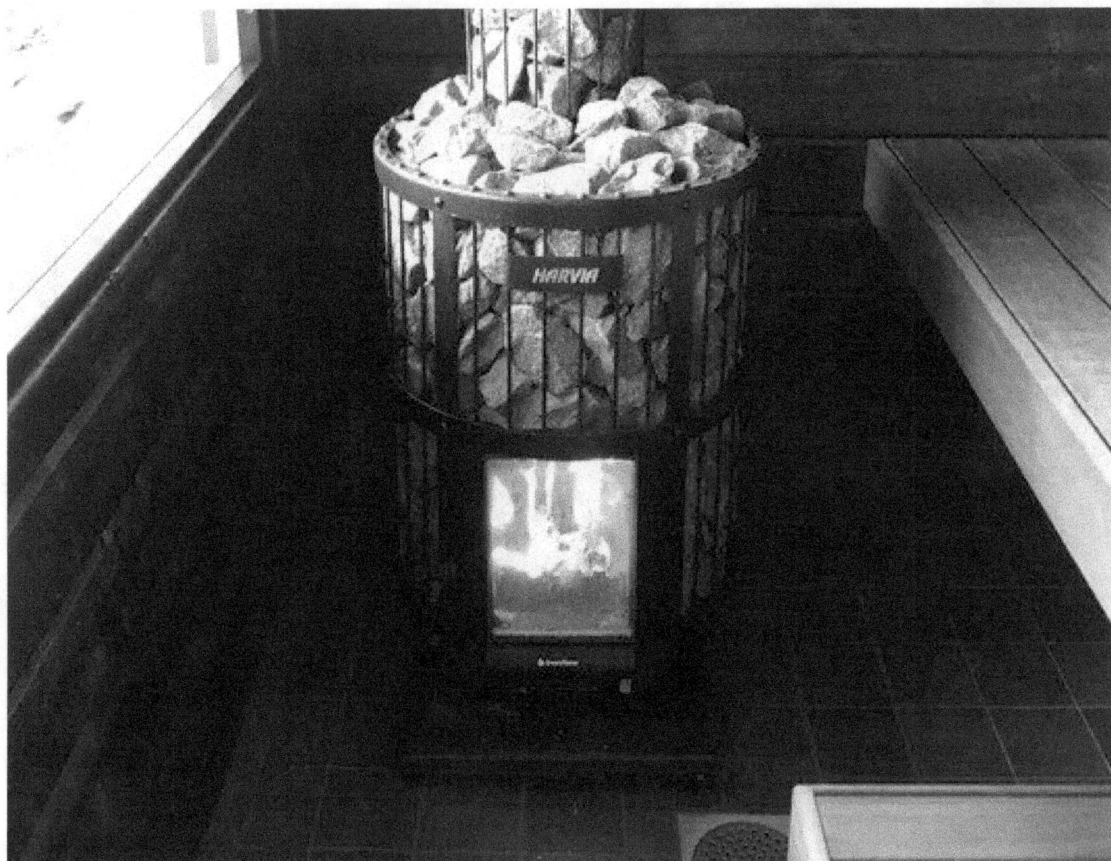

Harvia® sauna heater

THERMOTHERAPY: HEAT

FINNISH BATH (SAUNA)

DESCRIPTION

A small room with a heat source producing high temperature in order to make the occupants perspire. Originating in ancient Rome but popularized in Finland, this device for inducing detoxification became adopted by many naturopaths in the early 1950s as an adjunct or substitute for the moist **Russian bath**.

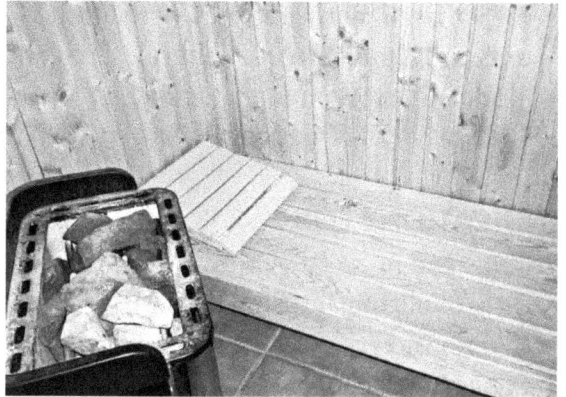

The Russian bath, in the form of a steam room or a steam cabinet, induces perspiration by the presence of hot steam. The sauna creates dry heat by distinction, by the use of rocks heated by wood, gas burners, or electric coils. Although users often throw water on the stones to make steam and increase the humidity of the sauna, the device is essentially a dry heat producer. Late 20th Century saunas have been manufactured using far **infrared** as their heat source, adding the claimed benefits of that modality (covered elsewhere here) to the obvious usefulness of induced sweating. The official Finnish sauna organizations have decried these infrared units as not true saunas. The heat derived is generally lower than traditional saunas, but has made it more palatable for the masses.

Whether called saunas or Finnish baths, naturopathic clinics have incorporated this modality as an aid to detoxification that can serve as a stand-alone therapy that does not require the active participation of the doctor.

EQUIPMENT NEEDED

A two-person sauna can be incorporated into one's office or clinic for as little as $5-7,000, if the heat source is far infrared.

EFFECTS AND PURPOSE
- The autonomic response to the hot environment is to try to cool the body by releasing sweat.
- Inducing perspiration will effect detoxification of morbid material in the soft tissues through the sweat glands.
- Vasodilation in the first 10 minutes causes increased vascular perfusion. With continued exposure, metabolic rate is raised and the oxidative process on toxins is increased. The easiest escape route at that point is through the pores of the skin.
- The heat activates heat shock proteins, which have been found to repair mutilated protein misfolding, present in Huntington's disease, Parkinson's disease, polyneuropathy, amyloid cardiomyopathy, and other amyloid conditions.
- Far infrared rays are known to reduce pain, accelerate skin healing, lower blood pressure, increase peripheral circulation, benefit chronic kidney disease, and modulate autoimmune responses. Their use in full-body saunas is well known today. They are in the frequency range of 2000 to 3,000 nanometers.

INDICATIONS FOR USE
- Colds and flu
- Drug or alcohol intoxication
- Hypotension
- Congestive headache
- Gout
- Sinusitis
- Insomnia
- Anxiety
- Prophylaxis against illness
- Recovery from endurance exercise

CONTRAINDICATIONS
- Heart disease
- Hypertension
- Peripheral vascular disease
- Anemia
- Weakness
- Cachexia

PRECAUTIONS
- Contact lenses and jewelry must be removed before entering.
- Patients should always be monitored when placed in any heated environment.
- Patients taking diuretics should take care to be well hydrated before taking a sauna.

- The heat is always greatest the closest one is to the stove or heating unit, but the heat also rises and collects at the upper corners also (higher benches are hotter, lower benches are cooler). Patients need to be advised of this. Children should sit on lower benches.

ADVANTAGES
- Mostly "hands off" therapy for the doctor

DISADVANTAGES
- Cost of purchase and installation
- Because the head is included in the sauna, there is a limit to how much the patient can stand, given that the dry heated air must also be breathed.

INSTRUCTIONS
1. Always check equipment first. Heat unit must be turned on at least 10 minutes before using.
2. Explain the procedure to the patient. Have patient remove all jewelry and contact lenses. Provide several towels. Have a changing area for the patient to disrobe before entering the sauna.
3. Dry brushing the skin before the sauna clears dead skin cells, better clearing the path for the elimination of toxic debris.
4. First exposure to the sauna should last no more than 10 minutes.
5. Second and third saunas should be broken up into two 10-minute sessions, separated by a cooling off period and/or a cool water rubdown.
6. Future sessions are to tolerance, but never more than 30 minutes.

FREQUENCY OF TREATMENT
Chronic conditions should be treated once or twice a week.

REFERENCES
- Lehmann, et.al., Therapeutic Heat and Cold; Ed.3, 1982 Williams & Wilkins
- Krusen, F., Physical Medicine, 1941 W.B. Saunders Co.

THERMOTHERAPY: COLD

COLD PACKS

DESCRIPTION

Application of a very cold, but not necessarily moist, appliance to the skin with a layer of fabric protecting the skin.

Contemporary use of cold packs involves commercial preparations made of a plastic cover and silica gel. After being hydrated, they are kept in a freezer 10ºF or lower. These packs are convenient because they are neat, mold over body parts well, and maintain a low temperature for a long period of time. However, they do not lower skin temperature as effectively as ice does, and do not produce anesthesia. Melting ice absorbs eighty times more heat than cold water. Naturopathic practice has always used ice for its cold packs but the modern ND may need to rely at least sometimes on the commercial packs. However, ice packs are not used for systemic thermotherapy or hydrotherapy in Naturopathy, as they are considered suppressive. They are included here as more or less an emergency measure for acute conditions.

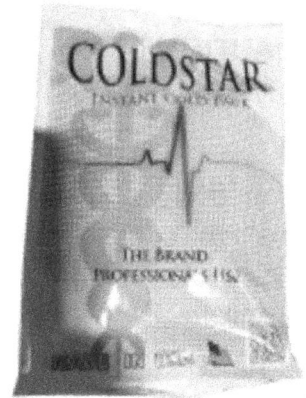

EQUIPMENT NEEDED
• Crushed ice
• Piece of flannel large enough to cover the target area
• Terry cloth towels (2)
• Plastic wrap
• Safety pins or other binders

EFFECTS AND PURPOSE
• Reduce inflammation
• Reduce swelling

19

- Draw blood away from site of congestion or hemorrhage

INDICATIONS FOR USE
- Headache or cerebral congestion
- Toothache and trauma from dental surgery
- Strains
- Sprains
- Epicondylitis (e.g., tennis elbow)
- Contusions
- Insect bites
- Acute bursitis
- Acute appendicitis

CONTRAINDICATIONS
- Acute asthma (on chest)
- Acute cystitis (over bladder)
- Patients or conditions aggravated by cold

PRECAUTIONS
Already discussed..

ADVANTAGES
- "Low tech"
- Fast response
- Pain relief without drugs

DISADVANTAGES
Need for refrigeration

INSTRUCTIONS
1. Spread towel #1 flat and spread an amount of crushed ice over an area the size of the body part under treatment. The ice should be one inch deep.
2. Fold and pin or otherwise fasten the towel so the ice stays contained.
3. Cover the target of treatment with the flannel.
4. Place ice pack on the flannel, over the target.
5. Place plastic wrap over the ice pack.
6. Place second towel over all and secure it (an elastic bandage can be used instead of a towel and pins).
7. Place another piece of plastic wrap over this to prevent leaking.
8. Leave pack in place for at least 15 minutes (usually 20), but not more than 30.
9. Remove pack.

10. Check treated area for reaction
11. Cover with dry clothing. Can be repeated every 1-3 hours, as needed.

FREQUENCY OF TREATMENT

Can be repeated every 1-3 hours, as needed.

REFERENCES

- Michlovitz, S., Thermal Agents in Rehabilitation, 3rd Ed.; 1996 F.A. Davis Co.
- Johnson, A.C., Principles and Practice of Drugless Therapeutics; 3rd Ed., 1946 Chiropractic Educational Extension Bureau

THERMOTHERAPY: COLD

VAPOCOOLANT SPRAY

DESCRIPTION

A vapocoolant spray is a highly volatile liquid (historically fluoromethane or ethyl chloride) in a spray bottle or can. When sprayed over the skin surface, it produces immediate and powerful cooling by its rapid evaporation on contact with air. The spray nozzle is designed to project a fine stream. Institutional and governmental policy-making has forced a change in these products as such chemicals were placed on an "ozone-depleting" list and considered to be contributing to climate change. Gebauer Company, the premier manufacturer, acquiesced to the complaints from environmentalists and the medical community and replaced its longtime product *Fluori-methane* with a non-ozone-depleting substitute, *Spray and Stretch®*. The name is suggested by the practice in manual therapy of spraying a target muscle with vapocoolant and then stretching it while under the analgesia it produces, commonly called "spray and stretch".

EQUIPMENT NEEDED

Bottle of vapocoolant spray
Toweling

EFFECTS AND PURPOSE

- Vapocoolant sprays rapidly diminish pain and tenderness, and render trigger points or painful zones more amenable to manual treatment.
- Useful for inactivating trigger points or *ah shi* points
- Allows painful muscle to be passively stretched

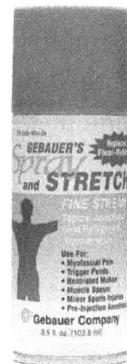

Gebauer's
Spray and Stretch

INDICATIONS FOR USE

- Muscle spasm
- Anesthetizing superficial tender spots
- Impaired myofascial function

CONTRAINDICATIONS
- Do not use on persons with poor circulation or insensitive skin.
- Do not use on open wounds or abraded skin.

PRECAUTIONS
- Do not spray in eyes.
- Over-spraying may cause frostbite.
- Freezing may alter skin pigmentation.
- If skin irritation develops, discontinue use.
- Spray and Stretch® is non-flammable, but older coolants like ethyl chloride and fluoromethane are flammable, so caution should be used to remove all sources of open flame and refrain from using any ignition products (piezoelectric stimulators, etc.).

ADVANTAGES
Lightweight, easy to use compliment to manual technics

DISADVANTAGES
Sale is typically limited to licensed healthcare providers; however, many massage schools sell as a sundry item for their students learning the spray and stretch technic.

INSTRUCTIONS
1. Tell patient what to expect. Observe skin condition and temperature of the target site.
2. Position patient for comfort and accessibility of the area to be treated. Make sure the rest of the body is warm.
3. If the face is in the treatment range, use some type of shield to protect the eyes and prevent inhalation.
4. Hold container nozzle down, two feet or so from the patient and spray at an angle.
5. Spray painful region in one direction only. Move the stream at a rate of four inches a second. Allow to evaporate completely before making the next sweep, being careful not to frost the skin.
6. Spray the entire target area along with adjacent areas. When treating trigger points, also treat the surrounding areas.
7. If patient has limited range of motion, passively move the body part while spraying, adding a slight stretch at the end of the range. Immediately after spraying, have the patient actively move the same part.
8. Process can be repeated if needed.
9. Inspect the skin after spraying.

FREQUENCY OF TREATMENT

Based on tolerance of the procedure and length of improvement after.

REFERENCES

- Hayes, K., *Manual for Physical Agents;* 4th Ed., 1984 Appleton & Lange
- A Practitioner's Guide to Gebauer's Pain Ease
- Johnson, A.C., *Principles and Practice of Drugless Therapeutics*; 3rd Ed., 1946 Chiropractic Educational Extension Bureau

4

HYDROTHERAPY

H

OVERVIEW

Although hydrotherapy has been used in conventional Physical Therapy, naturopaths raised it to a high art and historically used it—quite effectively—for organic and systemic conditions, not only musculoskeletal ones.

The true qualities that enable water to become a healing agent have to do with its thermal abilities. Water has the capacity to give off, and also absorb, large amounts of heat. It will carry heat to and away from the body twenty-five times faster than will air, for example. The thermal capacity of water, as well as its ability to conform to the irregular shapes of the different parts of the body, make it ideal for changing internal temperatures and manipulating blood circulation.

Blood tends to flow toward heat and away from cold. This phenomenon is important, for while a healthy person's blood will be drawn from all parts equally by such treatment, an ill person with vascular congestion in certain places will experience blood being drawn more strongly from those places with the greatest concentration. This advantage makes hydrotherapy especially effective for circulatory complaints.

Using hydrotherapy to change blood flow in a superficial artery will also cause changes in a deep artery from the same trunk, due to the phenomenon of collateral circulation. Thus, the effects of water applied at the surface of the skin can reach deep-seated problems. Also, arterial reflexes cause the reverse to occur: application of heat or cold to an artery will result in changes in the smaller and more superficial vessels branching off from it. This last is a great practical advantage in that the application need not be at a site where it would not be tolerated (due to a skin rash, burn or ulceration, etc.)

Another neurovascular phenomenon of which hydrotherapy takes advantage is the spinal cord reflex. Because bilateral structures are paired through the spinal cord, action on one can be taken by applying treatment to the other. This is of practical value when, for example, a limb is inaccessible due to being bandaged or splinted. The opposite limb can be treated to effect changes in the injured one. Temperature, duration, and timing of the hydrotherapy determine to a large extent the effects of the treatment. Let us look at these variables:

METABOLIC EFFECTS OF HEAT:
- Increased Carbon dioxide excretion
- Increased Oxygen absorption
- Increased serum glucose
- Decreased peripheral red and white blood cell counts
- Decreased tissue tone

METABOLIC EFFECTS OF SHORT COLD:
- Greatly increased Carbon dioxide excretion
- Greatly increased Oxygen absorption
- Increased nitrogen absorption and excretion
- Increased peripheral red and white blood cell counts
- Increased tissue tone
- Decreased serum glucose

Explanation of Phrases in Describing Hydrotherapy Procedures:

Application	Circulation	Temperature	Metabolism
Short hot	Stimulative	Lowered	Stimulative
Long hot	Very depressive	Increased	Very Stimulative
Short cold	Stimulative	Increased	Stimulative
Long cold	Depressive	Lowered	Depressive

Application	Duration
Short hot	< 5 minutes
Long hot	> 5 minutes
Short cold	< 1 minute
Long cold	> 1 minute

Temp.	Phrase	Effects
125°F	Dangerously hot	Can be injurious
111-124°F	Painfully hot	Intolerable
105-110°F	Very hot	Tolerable for short time
98-104°F	Hot	Tolerable, causing erythema
93-97°F	Warm / neutral	Comfortable or skin temp.
81-92°F	Tepid	Slightly below skin temp.
66-80°F	Cool	Produces "goose bumps"
55-65°F	Cold	Tolerable but uncomfortable
32-54°F	Very cold	Painfully cold

GENERAL RULES FOR HYDROTHERAPY

• Always explain to the patient what you are going to do.
• Treat the patient between or before, but never after, meals.
• Take the patient's temperature before and after treatment (below normal temp suggests increasing the hot portion of the treatment; high temp means the hot part should be decreased).
• Discontinue treatment at the first sign of any chilling (shivering will raise body temperature and negate the effects of the water).
• Compresses and cold sheet wraps should be covered with wool.
• Patient should rest after treatment and avoid becoming overheated or chilled.
• Cold applications are always preceded by hot.
• Cold applications are always short duration.
• End alternating hot and cold applications with cold (except in the case of extremity baths for arthritic patients, which end with hot).

CUTANEOUS REFLEXES (per Kellogg)

The correspondence of an area to be treated with hydrotherapy with the visceral target of the reflex action.

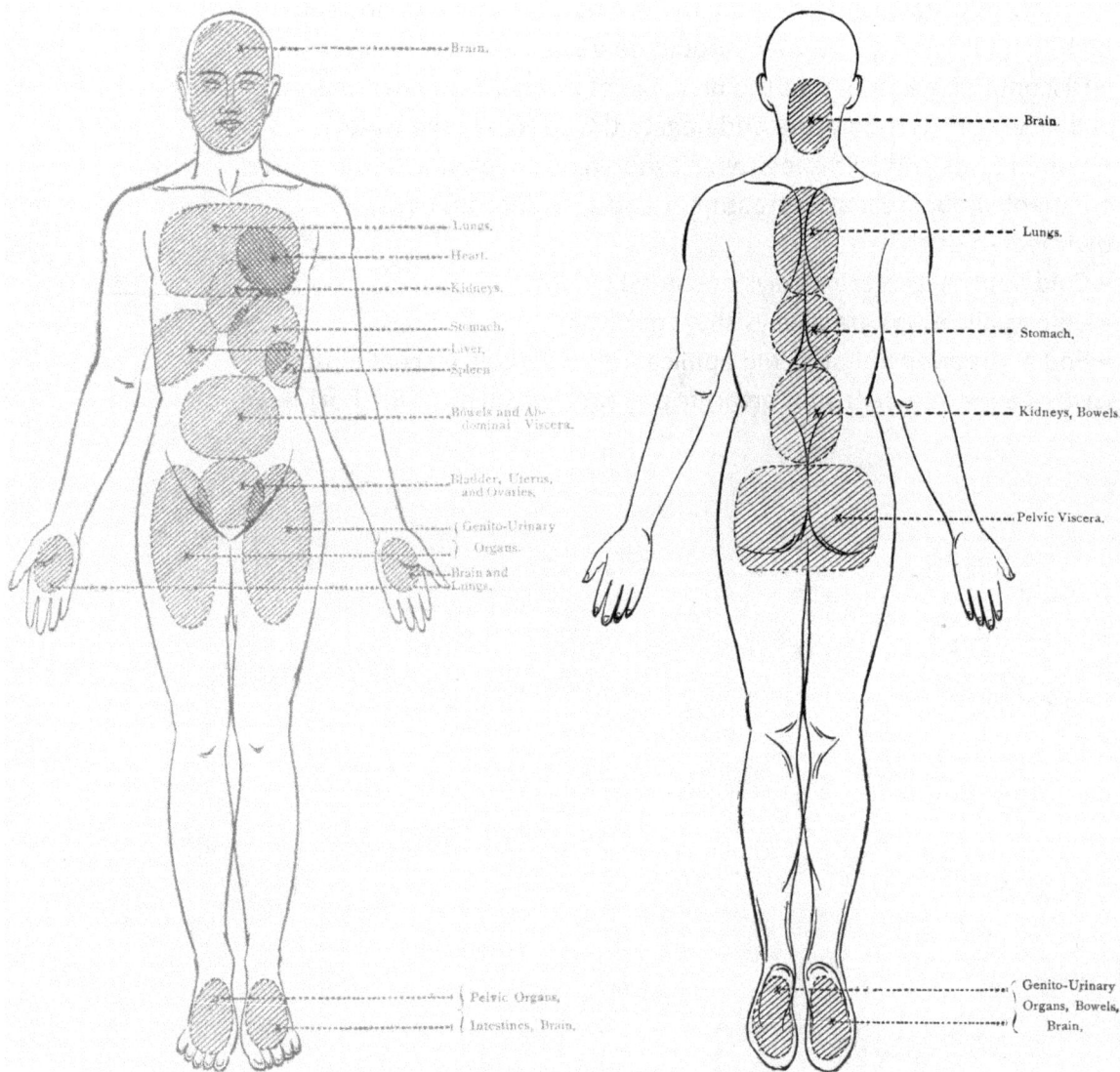

HYDROTHERAPY

HEATING COMPRESSES

H

DESCRIPTION
Compresses are pads of moist folded linen or other cloth, applied to the body with pressure. In Naturopathy, a heating compress, however, is **not** a hot compress. It is the application of a cold compress, applied to the affected part and covered with dry flannel. The area is warmed by the body by means of the increase in blood circulation it creates. **It is cold, used to provoke the body into warming it up.**

EQUIPMENT NEEDED
- Cotton cloth large enough for the area under treatment
- Flannel or wool cloth large enough to cover the cotton cloth
- Safety pins or other means of fastening the cloths into a compress
- Water-impervious sheets of various sizes (traditionally oilcloth, but plastic garbage bags work well)
- Towels and blankets
- Cold water

EFFECTS AND PURPOSE
The cold creates vasoconstriction, soon followed by vasodilation. This leads to warming of the tissues. Heat builds up inside the compress, creating further vasodilation. There are two ways to use a heating compress:
- If water-tight covering is used, the heat created is significantly higher, and *derivation* results (the drawing of blood and lymph from one area to another).
- If the impermeable covering is not used, the water slowly evaporates, gradually cooling and re-creating the same cycle again. The initial cooling is replaced once more by heating. The alternating of these cycles brings tone to the tissues, disperses congestion, and increases circulation.

INDICATIONS FOR USE
- Throat compress: Laryngitis, pharyngitis, tonsillitis, enlarged cervical lymph nodes
- Chest compress: Chest cold, early stage influenza, cough, asthma, pneumonia[1], chronic bronchitis, acute mastitis
- Abdominal compress: Poor digestive function, liver congestion, constipation, diarrhea, Crohn's disease, colitis, Irritable Bowel Syndrome
- Other local uses: Sprains, arthritic joints, boils, cellulitis

CONTRAINDICATIONS
- Local skin lesions that are easily irritated by moisture
- Very weak patients with poor reactive ability

PRECAUTIONS
Patient with low body temperature (<98ºF) should be warmed up before commencing.

ADVANTAGES
- "Low-tech" and easy to apply
- Can be taught to the patient for home use
- Can use socks, gloves, hats, underwear, etc. as compress material and coverings

DISADVANTAGES
Time consuming in a clinical setting.

INSTRUCTIONS
1. Explain to patient the procedure and its purpose.
2. Soak cold cotton compress in cold water and wring out.
3. Apply to the treatment target.
4. Apply water barrier covering if desired (advised if patient has poor circulation or is weak or chilly).
5. Wrap treated area snugly in dry wool or flannel to make it air-tight, but do not wrap so tightly that circulation is impeded.
6. Use pins or velcro fasteners to fasten the wrap.
7. Keep compress on:
   - overnight, or
   - until dry, or
   - For several hours, after which you can remove it, dry the skin, and replace with a new compress

---

[1] If the fever is higher than 103°F, change compress every 30 minutes.

FREQUENCY OF TREATMENT

Until the desired therapeutic effect is gained. A long series of heating compresses can be made, but with one hour of rest between each application.

REFERENCES

- Boyle, W., Saine, A., *Lectures in Naturopathic Hydrotherapy*,1988 Buckeye Naturopathic Press
- Dail C., Thomas, C.; *Hydrotherapy*; 1989 TEACH Services
- Baruch, Simon; *An Epitome of Hydrotherapy*, 1950 Ed., W.B. Saunders
- Krusen, F., *Physical Medicine*, 1941 W.B. Saunders Co.
- Kellogg, *Rational Hydrotherapy*; 1903 F.A. Davis Co.

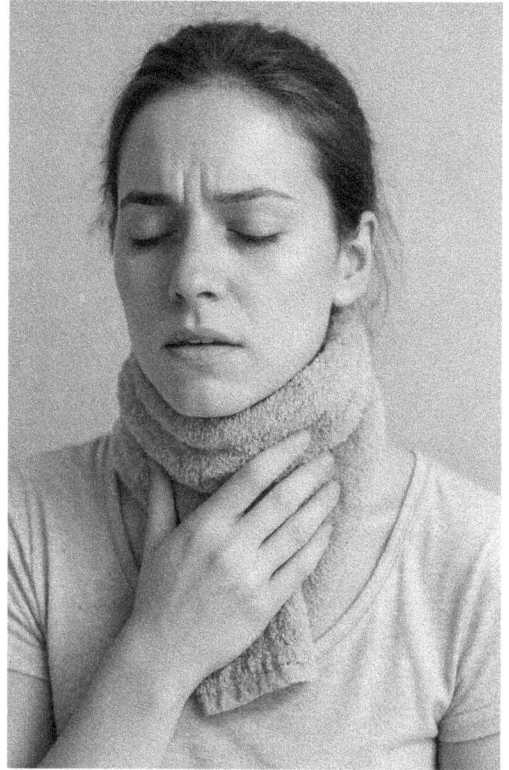

Heating compress for a sore throat

FOMENTATIONS

DESCRIPTION
Locally applied moist heat via a compress of wool, flannel, or other material

EQUIPMENT NEEDED
- Treatment table
- Pillow
- Sheet
- Blanket
- Hot water bottle with 104ºF water inside
- Basin large enough for the feet, containing hot water (104ºF)
- Tub for fomentation water, very hot (140º to 212ºF)
- Thermometer (for basin)
- Oral thermometer
- Terry cloth mitt or hand towel
- Washcloths
- Towels
- Heavy rubber gloves for wringing out very hot material

EFFECTS AND PURPOSE
Relieve local pain, congestion, and inflammation

INDICATIONS FOR USE
Inflammation, congestion, pain, myospasm, chest colds, bronchitis, pleurisy, back pain, sciatica, intercostal neuralgia, renal colic, dysmenorrhea, cholecystitis, prostatitis

CONTRAINDICATIONS
- Any patient with impaired sensation or ability to communicate pain
- Chilly patient

- Hemorrhage
- Impaired peripheral circulation due to diabetes, etc.
- Buerger's disease
- Deep vein thrombosis
- Skin lesions
- Malignancy

PRECAUTIONS

- Monitor the patient's comfort. If the application becomes too hot, briefly remove, dry the skin, and re-apply, adding more insulating material.
- If used daily, protect patient's skin with cocoa butter or petroleum jelly

ADVANTAGES

- "Low-tech" and easy to apply
- Can be taught to the patient for home use

DISADVANTAGES

Time consuming in a clinical setting

INSTRUCTIONS

1. Explain procedure to patient
2. Cover table with open sheet and/or blanket
3. Take patient's oral temperature and pulse, and record
4. Give patient hot foot bath x 10 minutes
5. Disrobed patient lies supine on table; maintain foot warmth with hot water bottle
6. Wring out fomentation material (several thicknesses) in the very hot water
7. Insert fomentation into fomentation pack, or cover it with several layers of dry towels (if wrung very thoroughly, there may not be so much hot water remaining and therefore can be applied directly).
8. Put extra insulating material over bony prominences, if any
9. Apply fomentation to target area
10. Close the sheet and/or the blanket
11. Check the patient's reactions often. If the application becomes too hot, briefly remove, dry the skin, and re-apply, adding more insulating material.
12. Change fomentation every 3-10 minutes (between fomentations apply a brief cold compress)
13. When perspiration begins, apply a cold cloth to the forehead
14. Repeat fomentation 2-3 times
15. After last fomentation, give overall cold mitten friction (but not in cases of conditions worsened by cold—pleurisy, dysmenorrhea, some arthritis)
16. Wrap patient warmly and allow to rest for 30 minutes

Monitor patient's pulse and temperature. Temperature should not go above 104ºF, nor the pulse over 140 bpm.

FREQUENCY OF TREATMENT
Daily if needed

REFERENCES
- Hayes, K., *Manual for Physical Agents;* 4th Ed., 1984 Appleton & Lange
- Krusen, F., *Physical Medicine*, 1941 W.B. Saunders Co.

POULTICES

DESCRIPTION
A hot compress with a medicated substance added. Made from a heated, moist and soft mass of herbal or other material, applied directly to the skin and covered with layers of first cotton, then plastic, then wool. The medication can alternatively be applied between layers of just cotton cloth. An archaic term for poultice is *cataplasm.*

EQUIPMENT NEEDED
- *Materia medica* for poultice: powdered herbs, powdered charcoal, clay, flax seed, mustard, or other vegetable matter like shredded potato or carrot.
- Hot water; enough to make a paste out of the poultice material (unless shredded vegetables, which are already moist)
- Cotton or muslin cloth, large enough to cover target area
- Plastic wrap large enough to cover the cotton cloth
- Wool large enough to cover the plastic
- Safety pin, tape, or elastic bandage for fastening the poultice to the body
- Washcloth
- Towel
- Heavy rubber gloves for wringing out very hot material

EFFECTS AND PURPOSE
- Relieve local pain, congestion, and inflammation
- Fight infection
- Provide counter-irritation, such as in a mustard plaster

INDICATIONS FOR USE
Anything you would use a fomentation for, with the added benefit of a medicated substance.
- Wounds
- Local infections
- Localized inflammation
- Insect bits and stings
- Chemical poisons or other contaminants

CONTRAINDICATIONS
- Any condition made worse by the poultice, such as an abscess that the poultice causes a greater buildup of pus
- Any materials used that the patient is allergic to

PRECAUTIONS
- Charcoal, while an excellent detoxificant, should not be used for extended periods of time as it will adsorb nutrients as well as toxins.

ADVANTAGES
- "Low-tech" and easy to apply
- Can be taught to the patient for home use

DISADVANTAGES
More complex than more modern ways of applying a surface medication, but the results justify the extra effort

INSTRUCTIONS
1. Explain procedure to patient
2. Moisten the medicating material chosen with enough hot water to make a thick paste (pudding consistency)
3. Apply the paste to the thin cotton or muslin cloth quickly (to prevent cooling)
4. Place on target area
5. Cover with plastic sheet
6. Cover with wool cloth
7. Pin or tape in place and leave on for several hours or overnight
8. Remove poultice, rub ice or very cold wet cloth over the area (gently if there is an open wound)
9. Repeat if needed—but only a new poultice.

Flax seed meal and powdered charcoal, equal parts mixed in hot water, is a typical poultice *materia medica*.

FREQUENCY OF TREATMENT
Repeat as needed, but do not re-use same poultice.

REFERENCES
- Boyle, W., Saine, A., Lectures in Naturopathic Hydrotherapy,1988 Buckeye Naturopathic Press
- Dail C., Thomas, C.; *Hydrotherapy*; 1989 TEACH Services
- Kellogg, *Rational Hydrotherapy*; 1903 F.A. Davis Co.

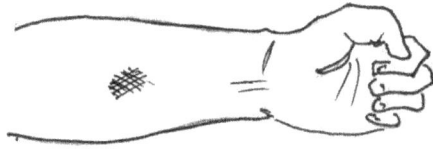

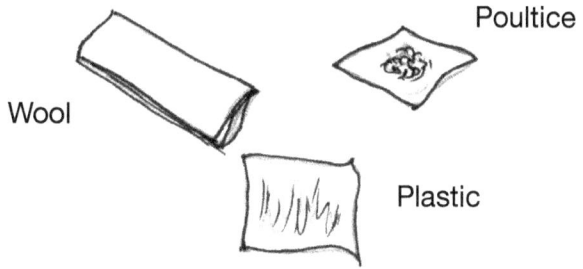

Poultice

Wool

Plastic

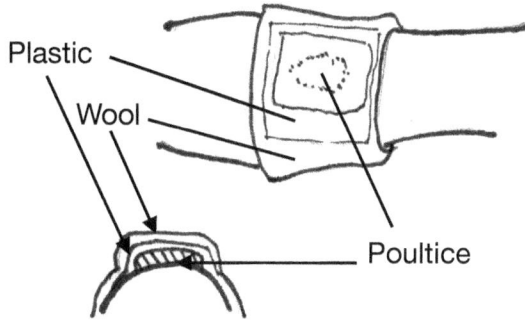

Plastic

Wool

Poultice

HYDROTHERAPY

HOT FOOT BATHS

DESCRIPTION
Immersion of the feet and ankles in water at 104ºF-110ºF for 10-30 minutes
Usually combined with **Hot Fomentation**, **Cold Mitten Friction, Wet Sheet Pack**, and **Salt Glow**.

EQUIPMENT NEEDED
- Source of hot water
- Tub large and deep enough (plastic bus pan or 5 gallon dish tub)
- Thermometer
- Rubber or plastic sheet to protect mattress, if performed in bed
- Terry cloth towel
- Blanket
- Washcloth
- Pitcher of ice water
- Ladle to add hot water

EFFECTS AND PURPOSE
- Creates local and reflex blood perfusion through the feet and derivation (drawing congested blood from other areas, including the brain
- Raises metabolic rate
- Increases white blood cell activity
- General warming of the body
- Aids in relaxation

INDICATIONS FOR USE
- Chest (pulmonary) congestion
- Pelvic congestion
- Amenorrhea
- Congestive headache
- Nosebleed

- Fatigue
- Preparation for cold treatments

CONTRAINDICATIONS
- Impaired sensation
- Peripheral vascular disease
- Arteriosclerosis
- Deep vein thrombosis
- Any other condition where circulation is poor in the legs and feet (diabetes, etc.)

PRECAUTIONS
Have treatment area organized and uncluttered to safeguard against accidents with hot water

ADVANTAGES
- "Low-tech" and easy to apply
- Can be taught to the patient for home use

DISADVANTAGES
Time consuming in a clinical setting

INSTRUCTIONS
1. Can be applied sitting or supine.
2. Properly drape patient first.
3. Make sure hot water is deep enough to cover the ankles.
4. Check with thermometer that the water has been brought up to 103º-104ºF.
5. Assist patient in placing feet in tub. Hold foot with your hand placed under patient's foot and into water first to make certain water is not too hot.
6. See that the drape (blanket) covers the tub.
7. Add hot water periodically, gradually reaching 110ºF. **Remove feet before adding hot water.** Check water temperature before replacing patient's feet in the water.
8. Continue for 10-30 minutes. Check patient reaction for perspiration.
9. If freely sweating, apply cold compress to the head.
10. At the end of treatment, pour cold/ice water over feet. Remove from tub, dry well, and cover feet. Avoid chilling the patient.
11. If patient is perspiring, give **Cold Mitten Friction** or an alcohol rub and dry skin afterward.

FREQUENCY OF TREATMENT

As needed

REFERENCES

- Boyle, W., Saine, A., *Lectures in Naturopathic Hydrotherapy*,1988 Buckeye Naturopathic Press
- Dail C., Thomas, C.; *Hydrotherapy*; 1989 TEACH Services
- Krusen, F., *Physical Medicine*, 1941 W.B. Saunders Co.
- Kellogg, *Rational Hydrotherapy*; 1903 F.A. Davis Co.

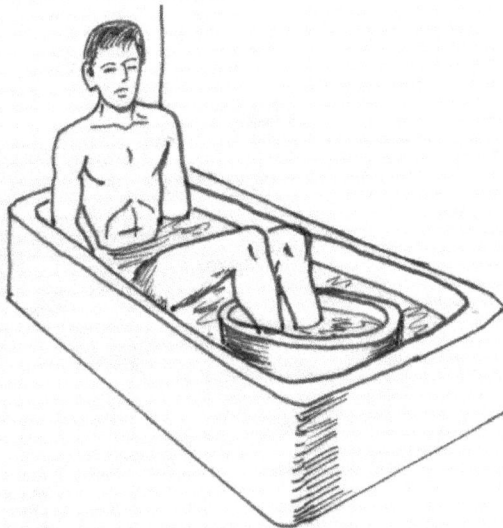

The hot foot bath can be combined with other hydrotherapy measures, such as tepid or cool bath to drive congested blood from the pelvic region to the heated feet.

46

HYDROTHERAPY

ALTERNATING (CONTRAST) BATHS

H

DESCRIPTION
A series of water immersion of the affected body part in alternating hot and cold water.

EQUIPMENT NEEDED
- Two containers large enough (and right shape) for the target body part to be covered with the water
- Source of hot water
- Ice for the cold bath and for head compress
- Drape sheet
- Terry cloth towels
- Pitcher to add or remove hot water, if needed
- Thermometer
- Cold compress for head

EFFECTS AND PURPOSE
- Alternate dilation and constriction of the blood vessels, causing fluids to be rapidly moved
- Increased blood perfusion locally and also reflexively
- Increased metabolism
- Increased oxygenation
- Increased phagocyte activity
- Accelerates healing response

INDICATIONS FOR USE
- Trauma (after 24 hours); strains, sprains, bruises, etc.
- Edema
- Impaired venous return
- Sluggish lymphatic drainage
- Cellulitis
- Indolent ulcers (bed sores, varicose ulcers, etc.)
- Infections

- Arthritis (rheumatoid and osteoarthritis)
- Congestive headaches (apply to feet)

CONTRAINDICATIONS
- Patients with diminished sensation
- Local malignancies
- Peripheral vascular disease
- Hemorrhage

PRECAUTIONS
- The stronger the contrast between the temperatures, the stronger the treatment.
- Monitor the pulse rate because there will be systemic effects, not simply local effects.
- "Long hot, short cold" is the principle.

ADVANTAGES
The contrast bath is one of the most powerful and rapid forms of hydrotherapy and produces change within one session, usually.

DISADVANTAGES
A little hard to coordinate but well worth the effort

INSTRUCTIONS
1. Assemble materials.
2. If treating infection, add hydrogen peroxide, betadyne, or other disinfectant to the water. If treating an uninfected wound, add *Calendula* success or tincture. Otherwise, just use plain water.
3. Position patient and containers so that a minimum of movement is needed to immerse the body part.
4. Make sure room is warm with no drafts.
5. Fill first container with in hot water 104ºF and place target body part in it for 3-4 minutes.
6. While the first immersion is going, fill the second container with cold water(or ice) water, 45ºF to 70ºF.
7. Place body part in the cold basin for 30 seconds.
8. Quickly add hot water to the hot basin to raise the temperature back to the original or slightly hotter temperature.
9. Place body part in the hot basin for another 3 minutes.
10. Alternate, long hot, short cold, for 4-6 alternations (number of alternations is variable but after 6-8, reactivity begins to lessen).

11. Every time you have a hot phase, the temperature should be a little higher, but never exceeding 110ºF. Never let the temperature of the hot phase be lower than the previous alternation.
12. Check pulse every five minutes. If pulse exceeds 120 bpm, apply cold compress to neck and ice bag to heart.
13. Finish with the cold phase. However, in rheumatoid arthritis cases, end with the hot phase.
14. Dry the skin thoroughly. Do not allow patient to become chilled.
15. Allow patient to rest for 30 minutes.

For body parts not anatomically suited for a basin, use soaked towels in the same way, covering with wool blanket for the redaction of each alternation.

FREQUENCY OF TREATMENT

To be determined by response, but any number of sessions are worthwhile

REFERENCES

- Michlovitz, S., *Thermal Agents in Rehabilitation*, 3rd Ed.; 1996 F.A. Davis Co.
- Boyle, W., Saine, A., *Lectures in Naturopathic Hydrotherapy*, 1988 Buckeye Naturopathic Press
- Hayes, K., *Manual for Physical Agents;* 4th Ed., 1984 Appleton & Lange
- Dail C., Thomas, C.; *Hydrotherapy*; 1989 TEACH Services
- Krusen, F., *Physical Medicine*, 1941 W.B. Saunders Co.
- Kellogg, *Rational Hydrotherapy*; 1903 F.A. Davis Co

HYDROTHERAPY

WET SHEET PACK

DESCRIPTION
The Wet Sheet Pack consists of wrapping the patient in a sheet that has been soaked in cold water, then wrapped in a second layer of blanket to seal in the reaction. The reaction initiates increased blood circulation and body warming. This is probably the second most powerful form of hydrotherapy (after **Constitutional Hydrotherapy**), and is sometimes called the "Universal West Sheet Pack", illustrating how global its effects and how various the indications for its use.

EQUIPMENT NEEDED
- Table or bed with pillow
- Materials for a **Hot Foot Bath**
- Washcloth for a **Cold Compress**
- Two wool blankets
- Two large cotton sheets
- Large basin or bucket of cold water (60-70ºF), 2-3 gallons
- One Terry cloth towel
- **Fomentation, Infrared lamp**, or hot water bottle

EFFECTS AND PURPOSE
- Using the temperature regulating function of the body to affect blood circulation
- Completing effects of fever by causing it to peak and then decline by the cooling caused by evaporation
- To induce a healing fever in an acute illness, if the immune response is not strong enough
- Relieve internal congestion
- Calm nervous tension

INDICATIONS FOR USE
- Heating phase: Common cold, influenza, bronchitis, gout, alcohol toxicity; also in measles or scarlet fever, to accelerate the eruptions and lessen the duration of
- Neutral phase: Restlessness, insomnia, agitation / mania, nervous exhaustion

• Cooling phase: Antipyretic action in already established fever
See chart at end of section.

CONTRAINDICATIONS
• Impaired circulation (diabetes, etc.)
• Severe presentation influenza
• Feeble or enervated patients
• Heating / sweating phase is contraindicated in anemia

PRECAUTIONS
Ensure that no loose places or air pockets are created in the wrapping. The neck and arms are the places to be well molded.

ADVANTAGES
• Powerful healing modality
• Low tech and easy to apply
• Flexible to be adjusted for widely varying conditions
• Can be used anywhere

DISADVANTAGES
Not as powerful as **Constitutional Hydrotherapy** due to the lack of accompanying electrotherapy

INSTRUCTIONS
1. Assemble materials needed.
2. Prepare table/bed (see illustration).
3. Patient must empty bladder first.
4. Pre-warm patient with Hot Foot Bath, Infrared lamp, or Fomentations
5. Fold first sheet in quarters lengthwise and arrange perpendicular across the bed with the end facing you hanging over the edge by about two feet, and the other, longer end hanging well over the opposite side (See illustration). It should overlap the bottom of the pillow.
6. Spread first blanket on bed leaving a few inches of the sheet visible at top, reversing the previous procedure with the sheet: This time make the overhang longer on your side and a shorter portion hanging over the opposite side.
7. Spread second blanket over the first but longer over the far edge and shorter over your side (opposite of first blanket's hang).
8. Fold second sheet in thirds lengthwise. Soak in cold water; wring out as dry as possible (usually requires two people, twisting at each end). Note: In fever cases, it should be less wrung out so that the sheet will draw more heat from the body.

9. Spread wet sheet on bed off-center, longer end toward you. It should fall two inches below the dry sheet showing at the top of the bed.
10. Have patient (thin cotton hospital gown for modesty) lie supine on the bed. The upper edge of the wet sheet should project three inches above the shoulders.
11. Have patient raise both arms and wrap wet sheet around body, under arms and tuck in all along the opposite side of the body. Below the hips, the sheet is tucked snugly around the leg of the close side, leaving the other leg uncovered.
12. Have patient lower the arms and hold them close to his sides while the other half of the sheet is pulled over and tucked in.
13. Fold down the top of the sheet over the shoulders so that the body is completely enclosed.
14. Draw the far edge of the blanket across the patient and tuck in the edge under the shoulder, torso, and around the legs. Also tuck over the far shoulder.
15. Grabbing the long end of the blanket, pull it to bring the other layers in close contact with the body and continue to wind it around his body, wrapping like a mummy. Fold the bottom around the feet and seal them in.
16. Now take the long end of the dry sheet and wrap around the shoulders, making a neat fold over each shoulder and tucked under. The object is to make the wrap airtight; also to protect the facial skin from the wool blankets
17. Duration of treatment depends on needed therapy (See **Phases and Indications**)

Note: Weak or nervous patients can be treated with the arms out of the wet pack; however, keep them inside the blanket. *Discontinue treatment if restlessness, headache, or vertigo occur.*

PREPARATION OF BED
(From Kellogg)

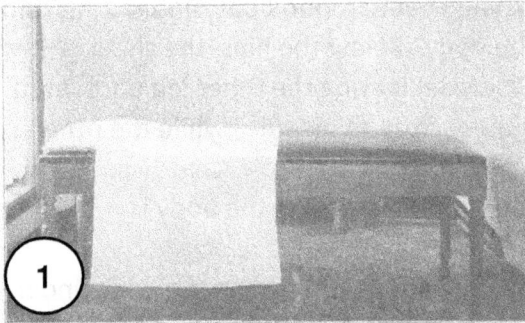

Fig. 74. WET-SHEET PACK — First Step (p. 601).

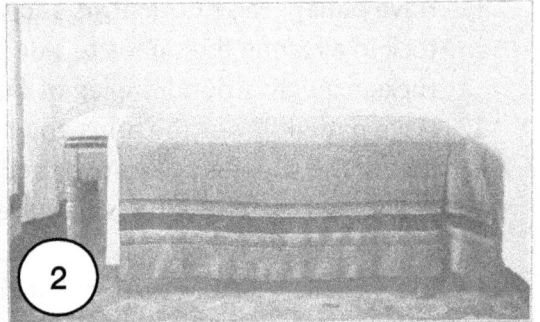

Fig. 75. WET-SHEET PACK — Second Step (p. 601).

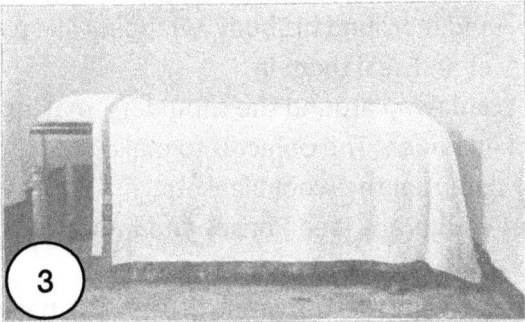

Fig. 76. WET-SHEET PACK — Third Step (p. 601).

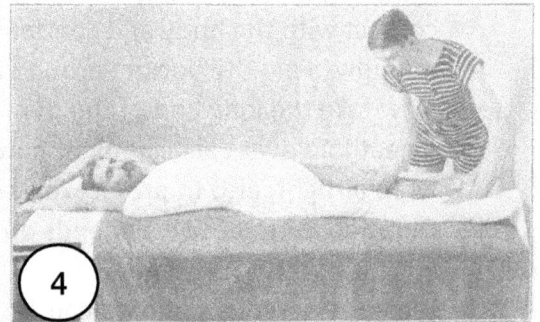

Fig. 77. WET-SHEET PACK — Fourth Step (p. 601).

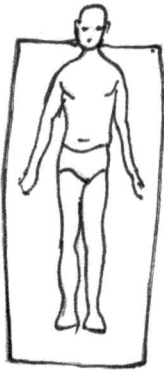

Step 10

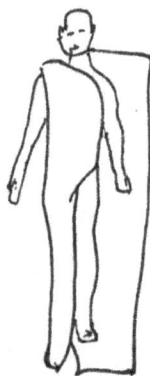

Step 11

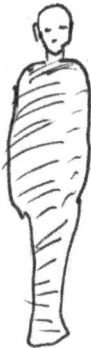

Step 14

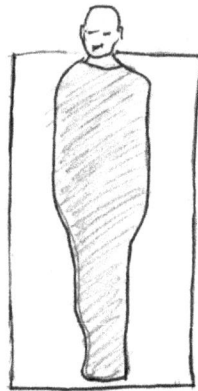

Step 15

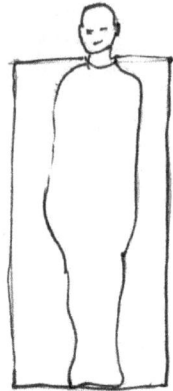

Step 16

WET SHEET PACK—PHASES AND INDICATIONS

I. Cooling	II. Neutral	III. Warming	IV. Sweating
Tonifying	Sedating	Activating	Detoxifying
Chilly to not chilly: 5-20 minutes	Not chilly to hot: 15-60 minutes	Hot to sweating: 30-60 minutes	Sweating to finish 1-2 hours (or longer)
Weakness; Fever; Anemia	Fever; Depression; Nervousness; Anxiety; Agitation; Hysteria; Delirium; Dementia; Neurasthenia; Epilepsy	Irritable Bowel Syndr.; Colitis; Maldigestion; Malabsorption; Crohn's disease; Acute nephritis; Liver congestion; Sinus congestion; Pneumonia; Constipation;	Environmental toxicity Substance abuse: drugs, alcohol, tobacco; Jaundice; Common cold; Influenza; Bronchitis; Periodic, prophylactic cleansing

FREQUENCY OF TREATMENT
As often as the case requires.

REFERENCES
- Boyle, W., Saine, A., *Lectures in Naturopathic Hydrotherapy,*1988 Buckeye Naturopathic Press
- Dail C., Thomas, C.; *Hydrotherapy*; 1989 TEACH Services
- Kellogg, *Rational Hydrotherapy*; 1903 F.A. Davis Co.

HYDROTHERAPY

H

COLD MITTEN FRICTION

DESCRIPTION
A cold water ablution coupled with friction from a Terry cloth towel or washcloth, loofah sponge, or a specially made mitt for the purpose. Performed either locally or full-body.

EQUIPMENT NEEDED
Any of the above-named implements.

EFFECTS AND PURPOSE
A strongly tonic treatment causing (initially) vasoconstriction, followed by the reaction of vasodilation, increasing the peripheral circulation while dispersing heat and reducing visceral congestion. Red and white blood cell activity is increased and metabolism is stimulated, accomplishing a central naturopathic healing principle: stimulate the breakdown of toxins and expedite their removal.

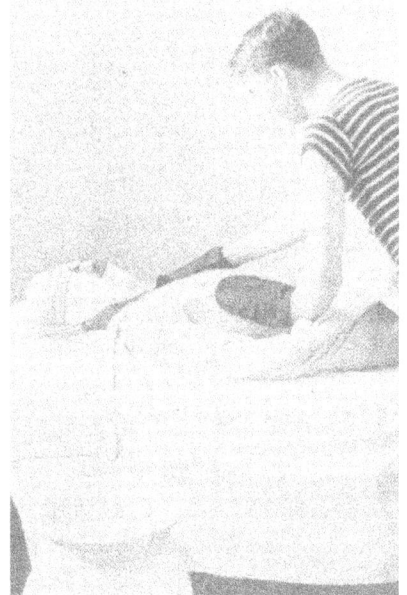

INDICATIONS FOR USE
- Prophylactic treatment to prevent acute illness (colds and flu, etc.)
- Sluggish peripheral circulation
- Anemia
- Fatigue
- Nervous exhaustion
- Depression
- Anorexia
- Fever
- As a finish to hot therapy, such as Phase IV **wet sheet pack**, **Finnish bath**, **Russian bath**, etc.

CONTRAINDICATIONS
- Chilly patient or intolerant of skin friction
- Skin lesions preventing friction

PRECAUTIONS
- The stronger the friction, the stronger the reaction.
- The rougher the mitt, the stronger the reaction.
- The colder the water, the stronger the reaction.
- The more often the mitt is dipped, the stronger the reaction.

ADVANTAGES
- "Low tech"
- Powerful

DISADVANTAGES
- Energy intensive

INSTRUCTIONS
1. Explain procedure to patient.
2. Ensure patient is warm before beginning.
3. Have patient disrobe and lie supine on the table under a blanket.
4. Pull back blanket to expose one arm, place towel under it.
5. Don mitt, or alternately, grasp washcloth (fold in half and wrap around fingers, holding in place with thumb).
6. Dip the mitt or washcloth in cold water and wring out (the weaker the patient, the drier).
7. Using back-and-forth friction, rubbing the fingers first, working up the arm to the shoulder and back down to the fingers. The skin should become pink.
8. Dry the arm using friction, and cover.
9. Re-dip the mitt or washcloth and wring.
10. Repeat process with other arm.
11. Expose the chest and abdomen but keep the arms covered.
12. Re-dip and wring the mitt or washcloth.
13. Use back-and-forth friction up the middle of the chest, across to the shoulder, and back down either side of the chest.
14. Repeat chest sequence, dry the area, and cover.
15. Re-dip and treat one leg in the same way, from toes to upper thigh, dry and re-cover.
16. Repeat procedure with the other leg.
17. Turn the patient over to the prone position.

18. Ask patient to raise arms to above head level. It may be necessary for comfort to place a pillow under the chest.
19. Keeping the arms and legs covered, expose the back and hips. Apply back-and-forth friction as before.
20. Dry and cover. Allow patient to rest for 30 minutes.

FREQUENCY OF TREATMENT

Once weekly if needed

REFERENCES

- Kellogg, J.H., *Rational Hydrotherapy*, F.A. Davis Co., 1903
- Boyle, W., and Saine, A., *Lectures in Naturopathic Hydrotherapy*, 1988 Buckeye Naturopathic Press
- Dail C., Thomas, C.; *Hydrotherapy*; 1989 TEACH Services

HYDROTHERAPY

SALT GLOW

DESCRIPTION
An application of salt to the skin, applied with friction.

Salt glow straddles the territory of mechanotherapy / massotherapy and that of hydrotherapy. Massotherapy being a common modality among earlier generations of naturopathic doctors, this method is still taught in many schools of massage therapy today, while it is included in the hydrotherapy curriculum in naturopathic schools. It is in a unique category because it is a tonic hydrotherapy that does not rely on temperature and therefore is not a thermotherapy.

EQUIPMENT NEEDED
- 2-4 pounds of coarsely ground rock salt or sea salt. Epsom salt can also be used.
- Sheet
- Towels
- Blanket
- Stool
- Basin large enough to fit around legs under stool
- **Hot foot bath** (instructions in that section in this book)
- Water to remove salt residue after (shower or tub is ideal, but can use sponge bath)

EFFECTS AND PURPOSE
The friction creates vasodilation and therefore increased blood perfusion, but unlike other modalities that do this, no temperature change occurs.
The mechanical irritation is coupled with a chemical irritation from the minerals, leading to increased activity of the sebaceous glands, a resultant increase in elimination of toxic debris from the skin, and heightened nerve activity.

INDICATIONS FOR USE
- Kidney disease
- Diabetes (only with intact skin)

- Chronic conditions, particularly with poor skin or poor reactivity
- Fatigue, weakness, neurasthenia
- Poor resistance to illness
- Frequent colds and acute illnesses
- Epilepsy
- Cancer (not directly over tumors)

CONTRAINDICATIONS

- Obviously, no friction over compromised skin areas; lesions, wounds, ulcers, etc.
- Eczema
- Delicate skin as found in Cushing's disease, etc.

PRECAUTIONS

- Observe carefully for any skin conditions that would be aggravated.
- Light-complexioned people will have less tolerance for the friction than dark-complexioned people.

ADVANTAGES

- "Low tech"
- Cheap materials

DISADVANTAGES

- Cleansing after the treatment can be laborious

INSTRUCTIONS

1. Assemble materials.
2. Place basin under stool.
3. Explain procedure to patient.
4. Seat disrobed patient on stool, draped with sheet and blanket over that.Note: procedure can be made with patient standing, in a large enough basin to both establish the hot foot bath and also catch the dripping from the procedure.
5. Place patient's feet in hot foot bath. .
6. Wet the salt to a sticky consistency.
7. Expose first region to be treated (arms first, working from fingers to shoulders).
8. Wet the skin of the region to be treated.
9. Take a handful of the salt and rub on the skin in a back-and-forth motion until the skin turns pinkish (or to tolerance).
10. Repeat process for next region to be treated are the legs, beginning with the toes.
11. Apply to chest.
12. Apply to abdomen.

13. Apply to back.
14. Apply to hips and buttocks.
15. Remove salt with sponge bath, spray, shower, or whatever method you have. Water should be cool but a comfortable temperature.
16. Rub the skin during the rinse.
17. Rub the skin again during the towel drying.
18. Ideally, the patient should rest for 30 minutes after procedure.

FREQUENCY OF TREATMENT
Once weekly usually suffices.

REFERENCES

- Kellogg, J.H., *Rational Hydrotherapy*, F.A. Davis Co., 1903
- Boyle, W., and Saine, A., *Lectures in Naturopathic Hydrotherapy*, 1988 Buckeye Naturopathic Press
- Dail, C., Thomas, C.; *Hydrotherapy*, 1989 TEACH Services

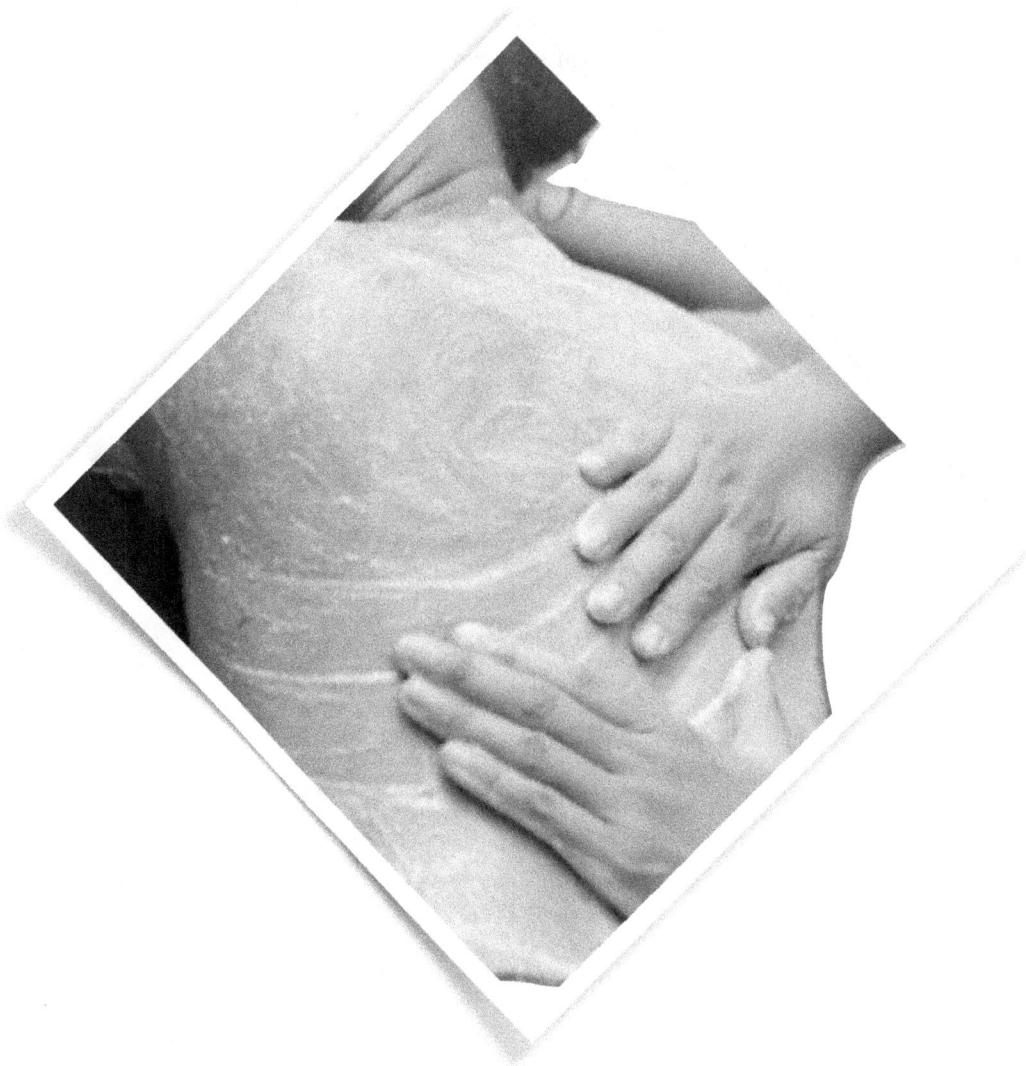

HYDROTHERAPY

LIGHTNING BATH
(*BLITZ GUSS*)

DESCRIPTION

This is an example of a mainstay of hydrotherapy in Naturopathy, one of the methods technically called a *douche:* a stream of water aimed at a part of the body. Variations include the Scotch Douche, the Fan Douche, and the Rain Douche. Today, most are familiar with the term douche only in its internal application; I.e., vaginally. Douche-type hydrotherapy measures are not seen as much today because they require a specially equipped room with tile walls, drains, and controlling equipment to regulate temperature and pressure of the water. But the *Blitz Guss,* or "Lightning Bath", is simple enough that it can be performed with a common garden hose. It is included here to encourage practitioners with the right physical plant to include it in their armamentarium.

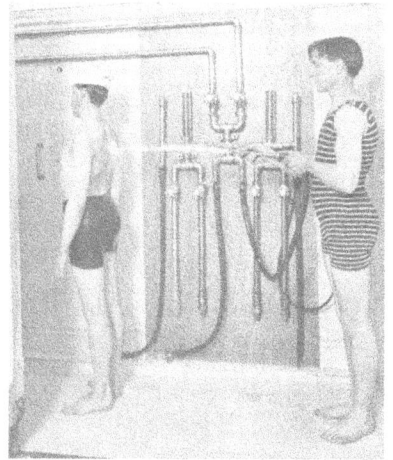

From Kellogg,
Rational Hydrotherapy

EQUIPMENT NEEDED
• Garden hose and spray nozzle
• Cold water (if hot water is also available, so much the better)
• Towels
• Warm environment

EFFECTS AND PURPOSE

The short cold causes vasoconstriction, which the body then reverses by dilating the blood vessels as it fights to re-establish warmth. This results in not only increased circulation, but up regulation of immune response, metabolism, nutritional uptake, and waste elimination pathways.

INDICATIONS FOR USE
- Anemia
- Fatigue, neurasthenia
- Visceral congestion
- Atonic conditions (atonic constipation, etc.)
- Maldigestion and dyspepsia
- Hypothyroidism
- Drug addiction

CONTRAINDICATIONS
- Acute inflammation
- Agitation, nervous irritability
- Acute flares of rheumatic conditions
- Nephritis
- Hepatitis
- Gastritis
- Hyperthyroidism
- Hypertension
- Arteriosclerosis
- Sciatica
- Skin eruptions or lesions

PRECAUTIONS
Do not direct stream at bony prominences in thin patients

ADVANTAGES
- No exotic equipment needed
- No particular skill needed—support staff can perform.

DISADVANTAGES
Temperature controlled environment with waterproof area needed.

INSTRUCTIONS
Water pressure should be 10-60 pounds per square inch.
If hot water is available, blend with the cold at first to begin and then make each repetition colder.
- Ensure that patient is warm before starting.
- Explain procedure to patient.
- Have disrobed patient stand , back to the operator, 10-20 feet away from the water source.

1. Apply water stream to the right foot first.
2. Quickly move the stream up the back of the leg to the right buttock.
3. Move stream back down the leg to the right foot again.
4. Apply to the left foot.
5. Quickly move the stream up the left leg to the buttock.
6. Continue stream across to the right buttock.
7. Move stream upward along right side of back to the right shoulder.
8. Move stream back down the back to the right buttock.
9. Move across to left buttock.
10. Move up along left side of back to the left shoulder.
11. Stop.
12. Repeat sequence 5-10 times.

The colder the water temperature, the faster the stream should be moved.
Each movement of the stream lasts 10-15 seconds ordinarily.

FREQUENCY OF TREATMENT
Determined by need.

REFERENCES

- Boyle, W., and Saine, A., *Lectures in Naturopathic Hydrotherapy;* 1988 Buckeye Naturopathic Press
- Baruch, Simon; *An Epitome of Hydrotherapy*, 1950 Ed., W.B. Saunders
- Krusen, F., *Physical Medicine*, 1941 W.B. Saunders Co.
- Kellogg, J.H., *Rational Hydrotherapy;* 1903 F.A. Davis Co.

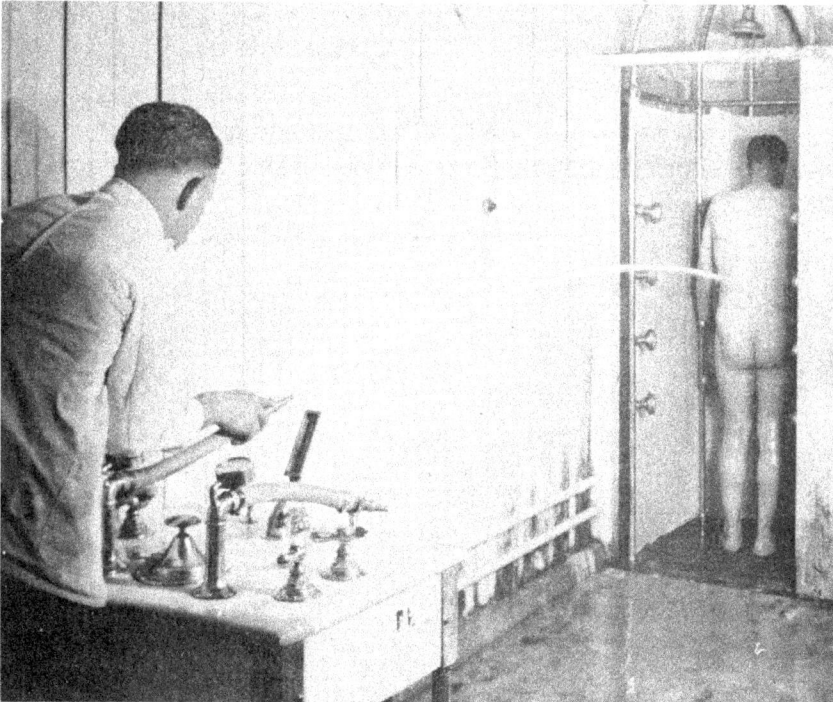

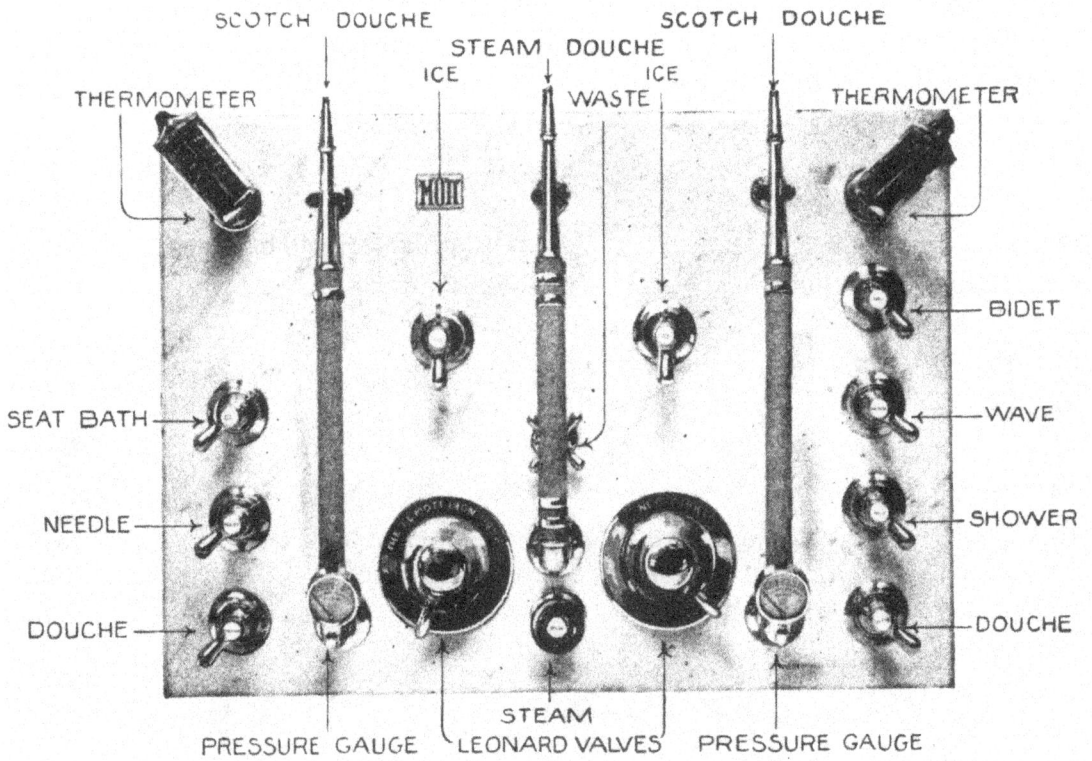

Design of douche table, designed by Penfrase and manufactured by J.L. Mott Co., as recommended by Baruch in his classic work, *Epitome of Hydrotherapy.*

HYDROTHERAPY

EXTREMITY GUSH

DESCRIPTION

The "gush" in the name is technically called an *affusion*; pouring a stream of water on a body part for therapeutic purposes. The arms or legs are treated by this method. It is effective for any local problem of the arm or leg, but the reflex effects of the gush are remarkable. The Arm Gush and the Knee Gush are described here.

EQUIPMENT NEEDED
- Source of cold water
- Hose or pitcher to conduct the water along the limb
- Chair or stand of some sort to stabilize the body (see illustration). A pole stretched across a bathtub can be used.

EFFECTS AND PURPOSE

Because of its action on the vascular tissues, the arm gush has a powerful reflex effect on circulatory problems, such as cold hands, writer's cramp, carpal tunnel syndrome, and arthritic inflammations of the joints of the elbow, wrist, and hands. It also can exert an influence over a greater distance; upper respiratory conditions such as sinus congestion, have responded to the powerful drainage effects caused by cold water over the arms, as well as dizziness and loss of sensation in the face and head. It is effective for draining the head and neck of stagnant fluids and has even helped reduce goiter. But the most dramatic benefit of the Arm Gush is in heart conditions; particularly valve dysfunctions, arrhythmia, myocarditis, and decreased ejection fraction such is found in congestive heart failure. The Arm Gush increases the strength of the muscle contractions, strengthening the heart's action in a safe way without resorting to cardiac stimulants.

The Knee Gush, because of its action on the circulation, has a reflex effect on the abdominal organs—liver, stomach, intestines, ovaries, etc. It also can exert an influence over a greater distance; lung and bronchial conditions, as well as sinus congestion, have

69

responded to the powerful drainage effects caused by cold water over the legs. It is also beneficial for chronically cold feet.

INDICATIONS FOR USE
Arm Gush:
- Poor circulation in the arms or hands
- Rheumatic joint problems of hands, wrists, or elbows
- Upper respiratory conditions (sinusitis, etc.)
- Vertigo
- Cardiac affections (dysrhythmia, congestive heart failure, myocarditis, valve dysfunction)

Knee Gush:
- Leg and foot joint affections
- Poor circulation and insufficient venous return
- Inflammation of the gastrointestinal tract
- Inflammation of the liver
- Inflammation of the ovaries
- Bronchial and lung conditions

CONTRAINDICATIONS
Skin conditions aggravated by moisture

PRECAUTIONS
- Care should be taken that the patient does not lose balance while undergoing the procedure.
- Those with dizziness or high blood pressure who might not be able to take the bending-over posture may sit in a chair and lean to the left or right side while that arm is being treated, or sit on the edge of a bathtub for the procedure.

ADVANTAGES
- Simple to perform
- Minimal time to apply

DISADVANTAGES
- Clinical setting , as with other hydrotherapy procedures, must be able to accommodate the drainage of water used.

INSTRUCTIONS

Arm Gush

1. The upper body should be uncovered, and if a stand such as seen in the illustration is available, the patient stands behind and leans over it, using the supports to rest upon. A pole stretched lengthwise across a bathtub can be used if there is no stand. The subject can lean forward over the tub and grasp the pole in the center (this eliminates the need for completely disrobing), or stand inside the tub and bend forward to grip the pole, if the lower body can be uncovered.

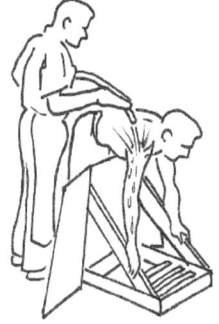

2. Direct a stream of cold water from a hose to trace the arm from hand to shoulder and back to hand, taking from 2-8 seconds to make the entire circuit. It begins at the right hand and the spray is carried slowly upwards to the shoulder along the dorsal surface of the arm.

3. Pausing at the shoulder will allow the water to completely cover the arm as it drains downward. The appearance should be as though the arm is covered with a film.

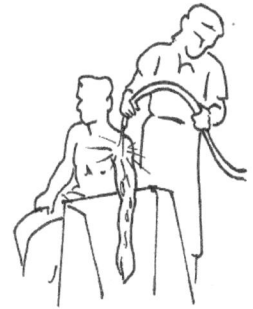

4. Now bring the water back the same way down the arm to the hand, and withdraw the stream.

5. Repeat the same procedure for the left arm.

6. Next, repeat the procedure beginning once again with the right hand, but this time the patient turns his hand outwards so that the flow of water will contact the palm, and make the water stream travel up the inside (volar surface) of the arm and back down again.

7. Treat the left arm the same way.

- The combined gushes—inside and outside surfaces—can be repeated once or twice a session.
- Those who are run down or anemic should have short arm gushes at first (2-3). Successive treatments can be 4-6, and then 8-10 gushes as the subject is strengthened.
- The ideal reaction is for the skin to become reddish in color and the subject to feel some internal warmth. If the skin turns blue, over-treatment has occurred.

Knee Gush

1. The legs are uncovered and a stream of cold water is directed by hose or water jet from the rear of the right foot to the toes, then back to the heel and up

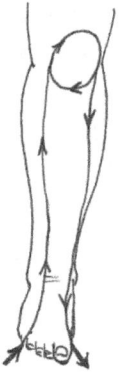
Front of leg

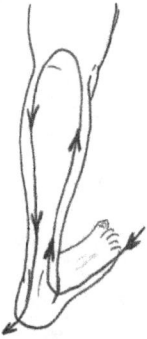
Outside of leg

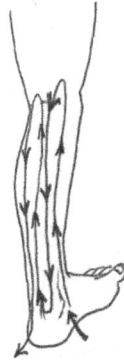
Inside of leg

along the calf, stopping above the hollow of the knee. The stream is kept there for a time, insuring that the posterior lower thigh above the popliteal space is covered evenly by the water.

2.Now the jet of water is directed downwards along the medial leg to the heel again. The process should take 3-10 seconds total.

3.Repeat the sequence for the left foot and leg.

4.Next treat the anterior leg in a similar manner. Start with the right foot, raising the stream up the lateral surface of the leg to the knee, where it remains for awhile. The water should also cover the lower thigh above the knee. Then descend by way of the medial surface of the leg, back to the foot (Avoid applying to the front surface of the shinbone; the muscular areas are what are to be treated).

5.Now switch to the other leg and repeat. Once again, the speed of the hose's movement is about 3-10 seconds to make the circuit up and down one leg.

•This constitutes one knee gush. Several are typically applied in a session.

FREQUENCY OF TREATMENT

As the case demands.

REFERENCES

- Krusen, F., *Physical Medicine*, 1941 W.B. Saunders Co.
- Kellogg, J.H., *Rational Hydrotherapy*, 1903 F.A. Davis Co.,
- Kneipp, S., *My Water Cure;* 1896 Benedict Lust Pub. Co.,

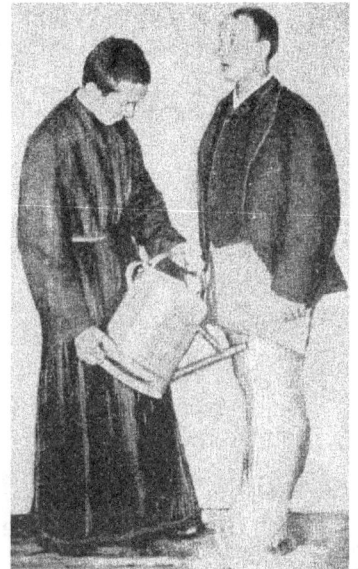
A watering can used for the knee gush, as per Kneipp. Certainly a low-cost alternative.

HYDROTHERAPY

RUSSIAN BATH

DESCRIPTION
A Russian Bath is simply a steam bath with the head excluded. A steam bath that does include the head was once referred to in the USA as a "Turkish bath", a term now out of date but nonetheless causes confusion.

EQUIPMENT NEEDED
Commercially made steam cabinet, or:
- A chair (an old wood or canvas chair is best).
- A sheet or plastic cover that can reach from the patient's neck down to the feet like a tent.
- Basin for **hot foot bath**.
- Tea kettle or other steam-generating device placed under the chair.
- 3 towels
- **Cold compress**
- Ice bag
- Watch or clock with second hand
- Drinking glass of room temperature water

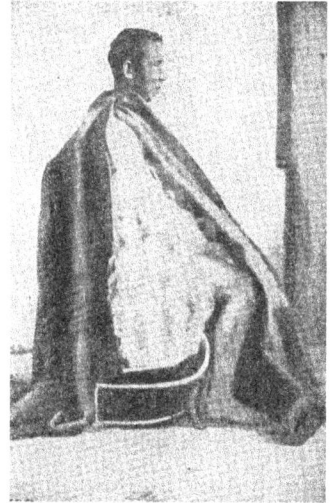

EFFECTS AND PURPOSE
- Raises body temperature, inducing perspiration
- Initiates detoxification
- Increases metabolism
- Increases pulse rate
- Increases blood pressure
- Increases peripheral circulation
- Increases circulating leukocytes in the blood

INDICATIONS FOR USE

- Colds and flu
- Drug or alcohol intoxication
- Hypotension
- Gout
- Sinusitis
- Insomnia
- Anxiety
- Prophylaxis against illness

CONTRAINDICATIONS

- Emaciation
- Anemia
- Advanced arteriosclerosis
- High blood pressure
- Valvular heart disease
- Diabetes
- Bleeding tendency

PRECAUTIONS

Discontinue if patient becomes faint.

ADVANTAGES

Effective treatment can be given even with homemade equipment.

DISADVANTAGES

A busy practice may need a separate room for the rest phase after the bath.

INSTRUCTIONS

1. Heat kettle placed under chair with spout facing the <u>back</u> of chair.
2. Wrap patient in the sheet.
3. Ask patient to sit on chair.
4. Pre-warm patient with a hot foot bath (104ºF).
5. Remove sheet, place towel around the neck and shoulders.
6. Replace sheet or cover, covering the body from neck down like a tent, also covering the foot bath.
7. Place cold compress on head.
8. Check patient's pulse often. If it reaches 120 bpm, apply ice bag to the heart area.

9. Encourage patient to drink water freely to aid sweating and detoxification.
10. Tonic effect is reached in 5-10 minutes; sedative effect in 15-25 minutes.
11. Finish by having patient recline (warmly covered) for 30 minutes.

FREQUENCY OF TREATMENT
Once or twice weekly, depending on condition

REFERENCES
- Boyle, W., Saine, A., Lectures in Naturopathic Hydrotherapy,1988 Buckeye Naturopathic Press
- Krusen, F., *Physical Medicine*, 1941 W.B. Saunders Co.
- Kellogg, Rational Hydrotherapy; 1903 F.A. Davis Co
- Kneipp, S., My Water Cure; 1896 Benedict Lust Pub. Co.

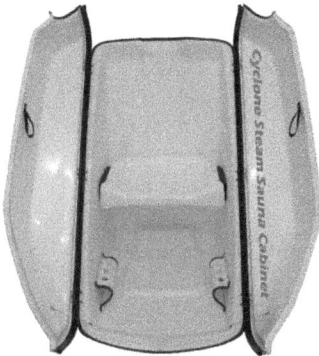

"Cyclone" cabinet made by
Longevity Resources
(ozone generator.com)

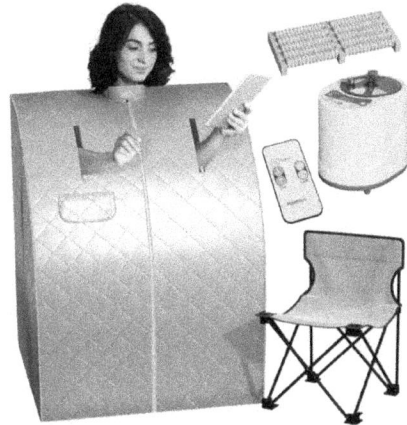

Moderately priced unit by
Anzzi
(anzzi.com)

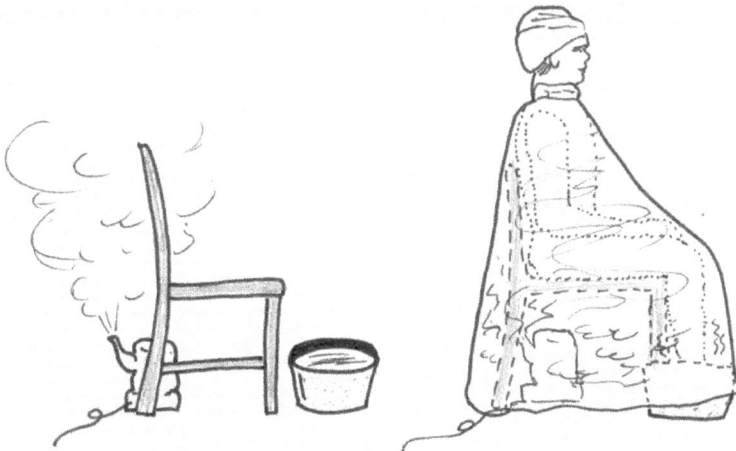

Homemade Russian Bath arrangement

HYDROTHERAPY

STEAM INHALATION

H

DESCRIPTION
A directed stream of water vapor from the steam from boiling water, inhaled through the nose and mouth.

EQUIPMENT NEEDED
Commercial steam inhaler, or:
- Heat source
- Tea kettle or other device for boiling water
- Sheet
- Umbrella
- Cone made of rolled up newspaper or magazine
- Aromatic medications as chosen

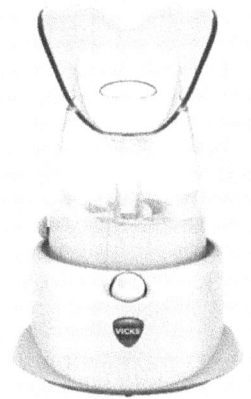
Vick's steam inhaler

EFFECTS AND PURPOSE
- Relief of congestion and inflammation of the mucous membranes of the nasal passages, sinuses, pharynx, and bronchi
- Moistening the membranes to alleviate sore throat
- Loosen secretions and allow discharge of toxic deposits from the lungs and throat
- Relieve bronchospasm (croup, asthma, etc.)
- Relieve coughing and relax airways
- Relieve dry mucous membranes

INDICATIONS FOR USE
- Cough
- Nasal / sinus congestion
- Bronchial irritation
- Spasmodic breathing
- Thick mucus in the respiratory tract

CONTRAINDICATIONS
- Aged and/or frail patients who may not be able to tolerate the heat
- Very young children

PRECAUTIONS
- Check patient frequently.
- Guard against burning.

ADVANTAGES
Uses the simplest of equipment and takes up almost no space

DISADVANTAGES
Probably best used as an at-home procedure and the naturopathic doctor should have ready a handout describing the process to be done at home.

INSTRUCTIONS
1. Fill basin with boiling water, enough to half-fill the sink or container
2. Add medicated oils if desired (eucalyptus oil, black seed oil (Nigella sativa), tincture of Asclepius tuberosa, etc.)
3. Use umbrella or large towel to cover steam source and your head in order to keep in the steam, or steam may be directed to nose and mouth with a tube of rolled-up newspaper paper
4. Breathe slowly and deeply for 15-30 minutes
5. Rest 30 minutes after treatment

Can be given after other procedures such as **hot fomentation** to the chest.

FREQUENCY OF TREATMENT
Can be performed up to 3 times a day.

REFERENCES
- Dail, C., Thomas, C.; *Hydrotherapy,* 1989 TEACH Services
- Kellogg, *Rational Hydrotherapy;* 1903 F.A. Davis Co
- Kneipp, S., *My Water Cure;* 1896 Benedict Lust Pub. Co.

HYDROTHERAPY

NEUTRAL BATH

DESCRIPTION

Full body immersion in slightly lower than skin temperature usually 94-97ºF. Its quieting effect is pronounced. Because it is neither hot nor cold, it does not produce an increase in metabolic activity as in hot baths, nor the reaction to cold as demonstrated in the other types of hydrotherapy.

EQUIPMENT NEEDED

- Bathtub (full size)
- Waterproof pillow
- Several towels
- Sheet
- Thermometer

EFFECTS AND PURPOSE

- The neutral bath's reputation for sedating agitated patients made it a mainstay therapy in psychiatric institutions for decades. It works its magic through a response to the neutral temperature by adjusting and equalizing the pressure throughout the vascular system. This reduces congestion, which in turn creates sedation (if there has been cerebral congestion, as there is in mania).
- Renal function is enhanced through both the regularization of blood flow through the tubules and the reflex action from the cutaneous stimulation.
- The neutral temperature reduces nervous input and creates a physiological zero point, allowing the nervous system to reset.

INDICATIONS FOR USE

- Hysteria
- Nervous exhaustion or neurasthenia
- Anxiety
- Mania

- Depression
- Insomnia
- Peripheral edema
- Drug withdrawal
- Hypertension
- Vascular conditions that cannot tolerate hot or cold hydrotherapy (arterioslcerosis, diabetes)
- Fever
- Toxemia of pregnancy
- Soothing of a healing crisis from other naturopathic treatment

CONTRAINDICATIONS
- Cardiac weakness with slow and feeble pulse
- Skin conditions aggravated by water, such as eczema

PRECAUTIONS
See to it that the tub is padded with towels on the bottom and where the head will rest, in order to make the experience restful.

ADVANTAGES
Can be used when either hot or cold is contraindicated.

DISADVANTAGES
Needs a bathtub and potentially a long time of application.

INSTRUCTIONS
1. Check tub water temperature for proper setting.
2. Assist patient into tub.
3. Place air pillow or folded towel under the head.
4. Cover exposed parts with a towel, or cover the entire tub with a sheet, held in place with weights or a board wide enough to straddle the tub..
5. Tell patient to relax and lie quietly.
6. Apply cold compress to the forehead if needed.
7. Check water temperature often and adjust when it is out of the desired temperature range by adding hot or cold.
8. Do not converse with the patients, except to reinforce the need for quiet.
9. Keep patient in tub for 15 minutes to 4 hours (longer times are used, but in excess of 4 hours, the skin is oiled with lanolin).
10. When assisting the patient to exit the tub, do not use friction to dry the skin, but gently pat with a towel.
11. Patient should rest for another 30 minutes after dressing.

FREQUENCY OF TREATMENT
According to the case.

REFERENCES
- Dail, C., Thomas, C.; *Hydrotherapy*, 1989 TEACH Services
- Baruch, Simon; *An Epitome of Hydrotherapy*, 1950 Ed., W.B. Saunders
- Johnson, A.C., *Principles and Practice of Drugless Therapeutics*; 3rd Ed., 1946 Chiropractic Educational Extension Bureau
- Michlovitz, S., *Thermal Agents in Rehabilitation*, 3rd Ed.; 1996 F.A. Davis Co.

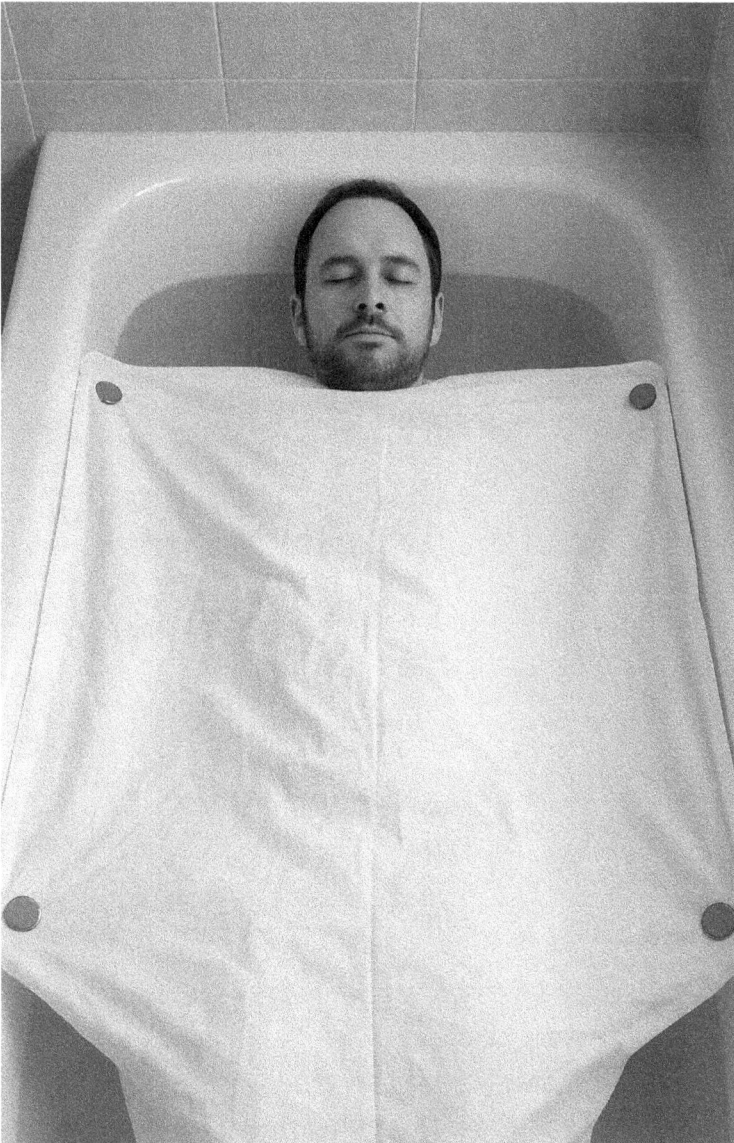

HYDROTHERAPY

BRAND BATH

DESCRIPTION
A bath of immersion in cold water, combined with vigorous rubbing of the skin, and then even colder water is poured onto the head and allowed to run down the back of the neck, then the immersion and rubbing is resumed, repeating the cycle.

EQUIPMENT NEEDED
- Bathtub
- Cold compress for the head
- Two or three one-gallon containers of cold (50ºF) water for pouring
- Towels for drying

EFFECTS AND PURPOSE
This method originated with Brand in the treatment of ongoing fevers, particularly Typhoid fever, for which it was markedly successful in the pre-antibiotic age. Roque and Wile demonstrated that the volume of typhoid toxin excreted by the body increased by a factor of five from the Brand Bath[2].
- Lowers body temperature
- Stimulates nervous system
- Increases respiratory activity
- Accelerates immune response
- Increases phagocytary power
- Increases the volume of leukocytes in the blood
- Increases muscle tone
- Slows the pulse
- Increases the contractile strength of the heart
- Reduces visceral congestion by increasing peripheral circulation
- Increases eliminative activity of the liver, kidneys, lymph, and the skin
- Increases oxidation to the point that the amount of oxygen in the bloodstream and the amount of carbon dioxide exhaled are nearly tripled in volume

---

[2] Baruch quoted statistics from a number of hospitals, the aggregate of which showed a reduction of mortality of 50% in typhoid cases.

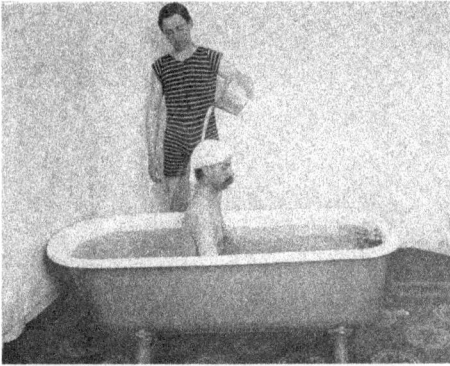
Brand Bath illustrated in Kellogg's
Rational Hydrotherapy.

INDICATIONS FOR USE
- Fever
- Systemic infection
- Sluggish elimination from liver, kidneys, skin, or lymphatic system
- Poor cardiac tone
- Poor blood cell formation
- Poor blood circulation

CONTRAINDICATIONS
Low blood pressure

PRECAUTIONS
In treating acute infection, the Brand Bath should not be used if the temperature is below 102ºF. Other procedures like the W**et Sheet Pack** or **Cold Mitten Friction** should be used.

ADVANTAGES
- No specialized equipment needed
- No hot water source needed
- One operator can perform in most cases

DISADVANTAGES
The discomfort of being plunged into cold water, although mitigated somewhat by the rubbing, is naturally unattractive to modern people. However, as a "heroic" measure in disease, particularly when antimicrobial therapy is not available or is ineffective, the Brand Bath could be the difference between life and death.

INSTRUCTIONS
1. Explain the process to the patient first, emphasizing the momentary nature of the cold and the role of the rubbing in lessening the cold.
2. Cool patient's head and face first with cold compresses with water of 50ºF.
3. Prepare bath with water at a temperature of 65-70ºF.
4. Fill several vessels (gallon volume) with cold water of 50ºF.
5. Place a towel soaked with ice water around patient's head and trailing down the back of the neck.
6. Conduct the patient into the tub quickly and immerse up to the neck. Shoulders should not be exposed.

7. Vigorously rub the patient's skin while submerged; shoulders, arms, chest, etc. for 2-3 minutes.
8. Have patient sit upright and operator pours 2 or 3 gallons of the prepared cold water on the covered head and allowed to run down the back of the neck.
9. Return the patient to a recumbent position and repeat the rubbing.
10. Patient remains in the bath for 10-20 minutes.
11. Help patient exit the bath quickly and wrap in a sheet, then cover with a blanket. The limbs can be rubbed through this covering. A hot foot bath or hot water bottle can be placed on the feet to further warm the patient.
12. The bath is usually repeated in 3 hours' time in acute infections

FREQUENCY OF TREATMENT
Case dependent.

REFERENCES
- Kellogg, J.H., *Rational Hydrotherapy*; 1903 F.A. Davis Co.
- Baruch, Simon; *An Epitome of Hydrotherapy;* 1950 Ed., W.B. Saunders
- Thorne, W.B.; T*he Shott Methods of the Treatment of Chronic Diseases of therapies of the Heart*, 5th Ed., 1906 Blakiston's Son & Co.

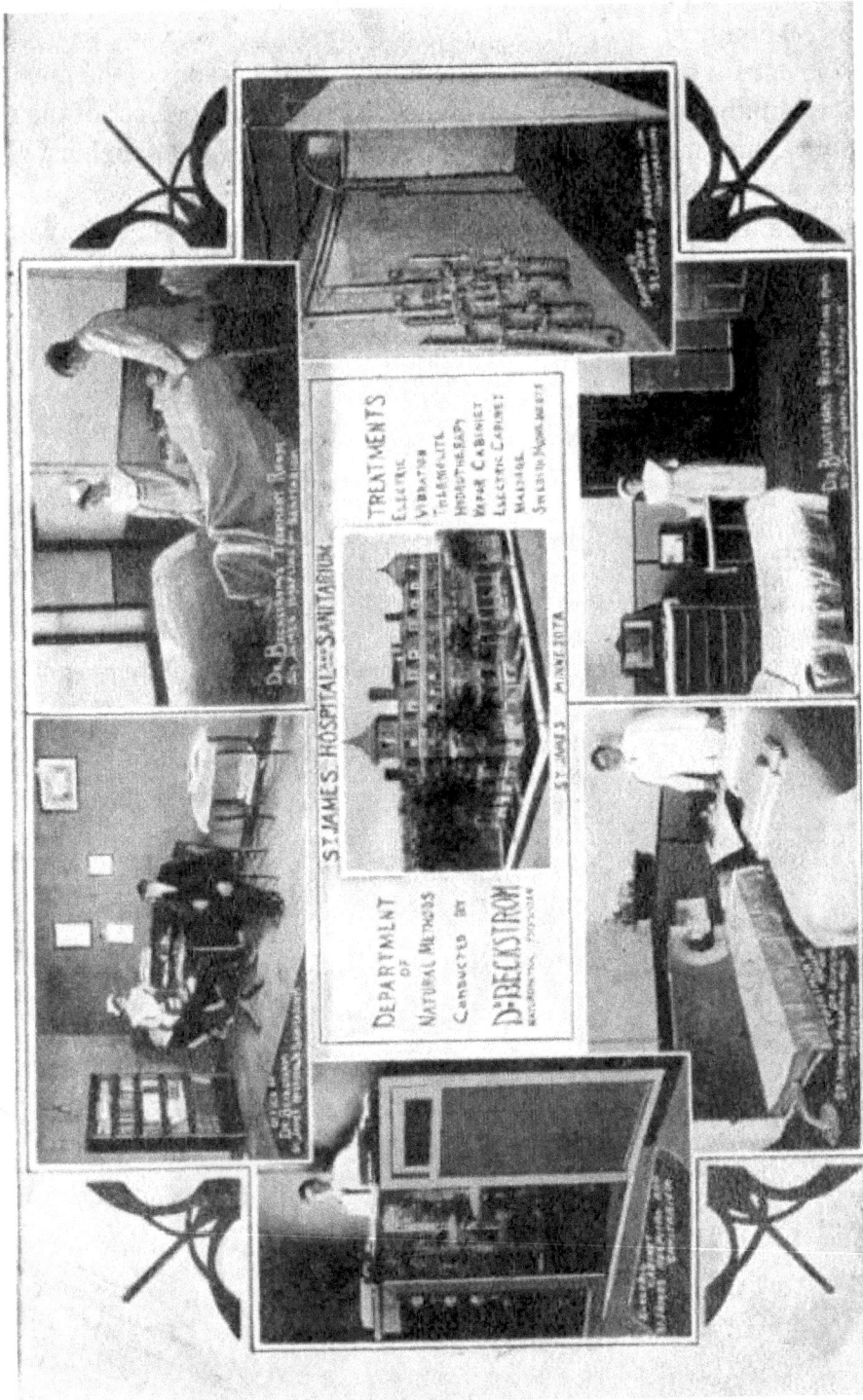

HYDROTHERAPY

EPSOM SALT BATH

H

DESCRIPTION
Immersion in a tub of hot water in which a quantity of Epsom salt (magnesium sulfate) has been dissolved.

EQUIPMENT NEEDED
• Bath tub
• Supply of Epsom salt

EFFECTS AND PURPOSE
The Epsom salt bath not only cleanses the skin of many of its impurities but it draws out a huge amount of urates and other waste products from the subdermal tissues. Carbon dioxide gas in the blood is rapidly reduced, increasing the oxygen concentration in the body. Carbonic acid and partially oxidized impurities are drawn out of the tissues by osmosis. Epsom salt being a magnesium salt, the properties of the magnesium are absorbed by the body as well, giving rapid relief of cramps or spasms. Irritation of the nerves is reduced dramatically by this bath.

INDICATIONS FOR USE
• General detoxification
• Sciatica and back pain
• Myalgia
• Neuralgia
• Neuritis
• Gout
• Rheumatoid arthritis
• Insomnia
• Nervousness

CONTRAINDICATIONS
• Very high blood pressure
• Pregnancy

PRECAUTIONS
- As carbonic acid is drawn out of the tissues by osmosis in this bath, no soap (a carbon-based substance) or soap residue should be present in the tub.
- Patients with diminished perception of heat should be monitored and the water temperature lower than usual.
- Patients who are weak or anemic should begin with a smaller quantity of Epsom salt (½ to 1 pound).

ADVANTAGES
- Little preparation needed
- Epsom salt is cheap and plentiful

DISADVANTAGES
- Tub needed
- Bath is continued for some time

INSTRUCTIONS
1. Rinse and wipe the tub to ensure that no residue of soap remains.
2. Cover the overflow valve so that the water level can reach the neck when reclining in the tub (wedging a piece of cloth into it usually works).
3. Line the bottom of the tub with some thick layers of towels for padding
4. Have patient drink 8 ounces of water before, during, and following the bath.
5. Fill the tub with water. It should ideally be three degrees warmer than body temperature, typically about 102º F.
6. As the tub fills, dissolve 2-4 lbs. of Epsom salt in the hot bath. The more that is used, the greater will be the action of the bath.
7. Have patient enter the bath. If this temperature is uncomfortable, make it a little cooler, then add more hot water once he has become accustomed to the temperature.
8. Immerse the body and cover abdomen, knees, or any body parts that stick out of the water with washcloths or towels saturated with the water. You want every part of the body covered with the solution but the head and face.
9. As the towels become cool, re-dip them in the bath and cover again.
10. Soak for 10-30 minutes, depending on patient's strength. The first time should be fairly short duration. As the detoxification progresses, longer times can be used.
11. Water should be drunk by the patient during and after.
12. Care must be taken when rising from bath so as to not to lose balance.

FREQUENCY OF TREATMENT
2-3 sessions a week (Note: Patient can be taught to perform at home)

REFERENCES

- Johnson, A.C., *Principles and Practice of Drugless Therapeutics*; 3rd Ed., 1946 Chiropractic Educational Extension Bureau
- Lake, T.T., *Treatment By Neuropathy and The Encyclopedia of Manipulative Therapeutics*, 1946

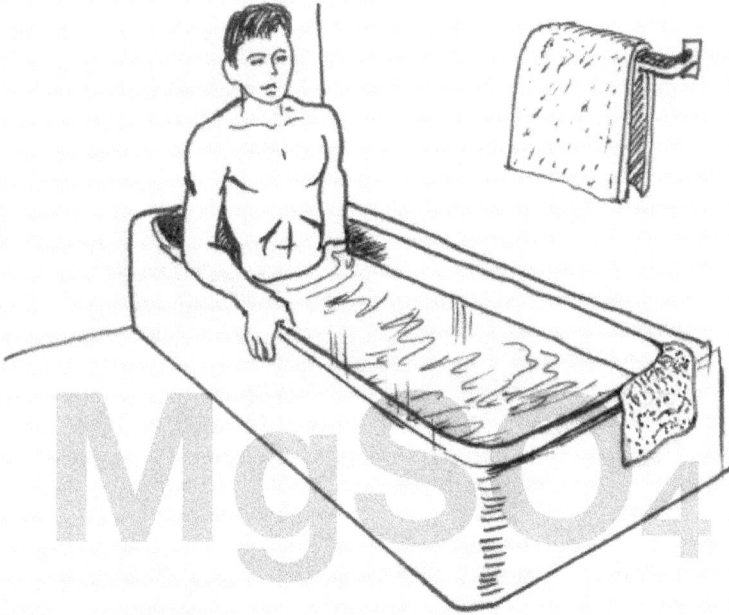

HYDROTHERAPY

CARBON DIOXIDE BATH

DESCRIPTION
Also historically referred to as the Nauheim Bath or the Schott Bath, the Carbon Dioxide Bath is a body immersion with elements added that produce carbon dioxide bubbles in the bath, with their resultant effects.

EQUIPMENT NEEDED
- Bath tub
- Blanket or other cover for tub.
- Fountain syringe (enema bag, or other dispenser with a variable spigot)
- 7 oz. bicarbonate of soda
- 4 pounds salt
- 12 oz. citric acid crystals

EFFECTS AND PURPOSE
- In a saline immersion, carbon dioxide is rapidly absorbed by the blood. There is direct stimulation of the unstriated muscle fibers of the heart, arteries, and arterioles. The resulting increase in blood flow prevents stasis in the vessels.
- The diminution of peripheral resistance lessens the burden on the heart.
- The heart diminishes in size due to the absence of excess blood in its cavities, and gains strength by having more room to contract.
- Respiration is enhanced by the CO_2, which is a stimulant to the respiratory center and increases the inspiratory volume and increases removal of venous blood.
- Astringent action on the skin but also creates a hyperemia that draws a large amount of circulation from the deeper vessels and lessens the strain on the heart.
- Absorbed CO_2 causes the left ventricle to more forcefully move blood to the periphery.
- The above create a training effect for the vasculature, which is effective despite such a short duration treatment.

INDICATIONS FOR USE
- Cardiovascular diseases
- Angina pectoris
- Hypertension
- Mitral insufficiency
- Arteriosclerosis
- Kidney disease
- Rheumatism / arthritis
- Nervous conditions and neurasthenia

CONTRAINDICATIONS
Any skin condition aggravated by turbulence of the water

PRECAUTIONS
If any flushing, headache, or excitement occurs, terminate the bath.

ADVANTAGES
- A tremendous non-pharmaceutical tool for cardiovascular diseases that are typically treated conventionally
- Short treatment time and clean up

DISADVANTAGES
Need for storage of quantities of mineral materials

INSTRUCTIONS
1. Assemble materials and explain procedure to patient.
2. Fill bath water at 95 ºF (usually 20 gallons water).
3. Dissolve 7 oz. bicarbonate of soda and 4 pounds salt in the bath. Note: Omit the salt in nervous conditions.
4. Dilute 12 oz. citric acid crystals. in 1 ½ pints water inside a fountain syringe or other dispenser with a variable spigot, hung above the bathtub.
5. Check and record patients pulse and place in the tub.
6. Once patient is in tub, release the diluted acid through the tube into the bottom of the tub. Small bubbles will form that will cover the patient's body.
7. Cover the tub with a blanket or other cover to trap the gases.
8. Patient's pulse usually becomes slower and stronger within 5-6 minutes.
9. Bath duration should be 7-8 minutes.
10. Bath should be given daily for 3 days. On the 3rd day, the temperature should be lowered one degree, and the duration increased by one minute from the previous day.

11. Skip 2 days and resume. Temperature of the bath water should be gradually lowered until it reaches 84 ºF. Also, duration should be gradually increased up to 20 minutes.
12. After each bath, the patient should be gently dried without much friction, and allowed to rest for 30-60 minutes.

A course of 10-12 treatments are sufficient for most cases, although the official course for Nauheim baths run to 21 sessions.

FREQUENCY OF TREATMENT
After the initial three sessions, every 3rd day or less frequently.

REFERENCES
- Baruch, Simon; *An Epitome of Hydrotherapy*, 1950 Ed., W.B. Saunders
- Thorne, W.B.; *The Shott Methods of the Treatment of Chronic Diseases of therapies of the Heart*, 5th Ed., 1906 Blakiston's Son & Co.

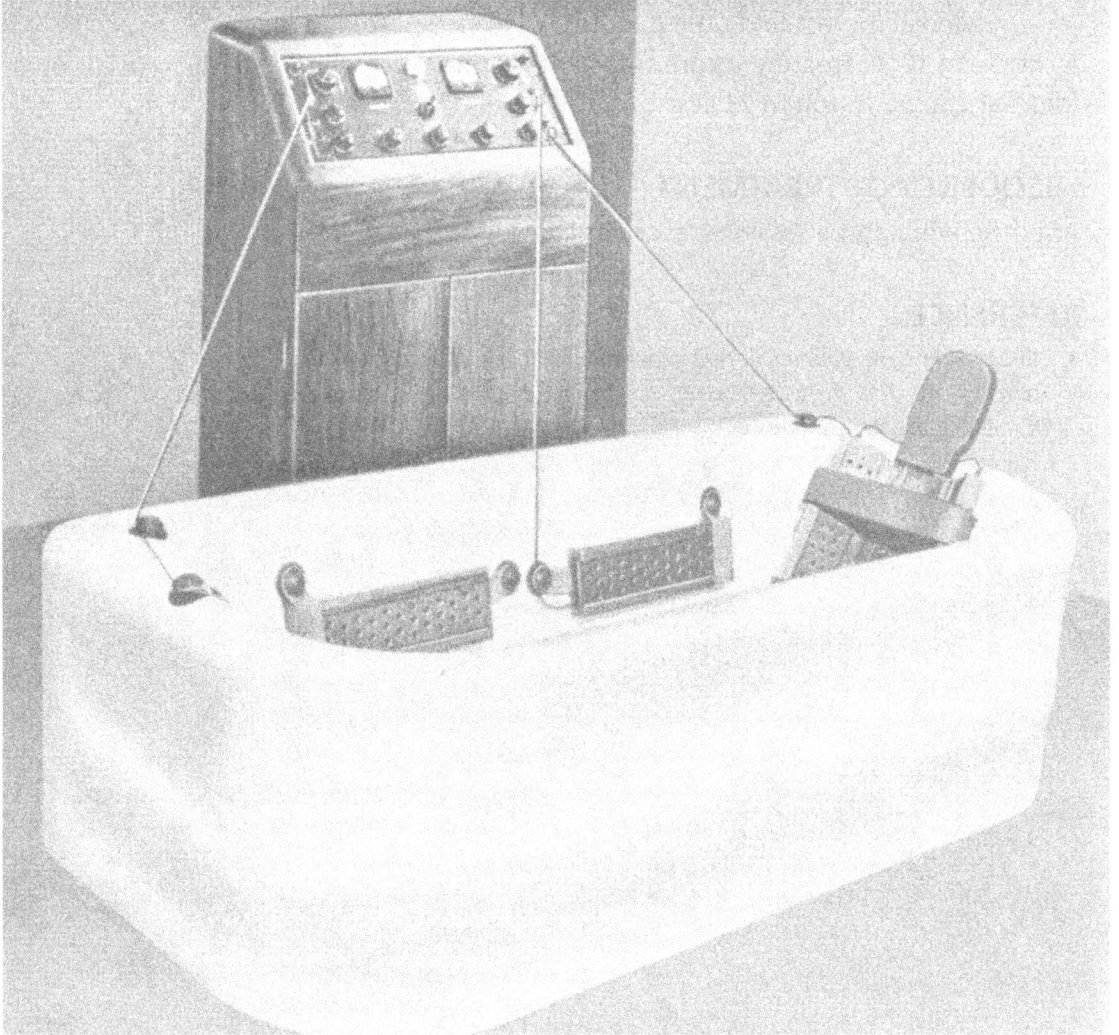

Tub manufactured by the Teca Corporation, for administering electrogalvanic baths. This is a hybrid hydrotherapy / electrotherapy method that uses the galvanic current to drive in medicinal compounds residing in herbs and/or minerals added to the water. See **Ionization** section for more details.

The Schnee Four Cell galvanic bath[3] may have disappeared from U.S. clinics, but it is still in use in European naturopathic facilities. This is another hybrid method linking hydrotherapy with electrotherapy, and at first glance it looks preposterous. Putting all four limbs in electrified water? It is easy to see how this was maligned as "quackery" by the medical establishment. Although the process uses low current from batteries and directs it from hand to foot, it was derided as "useless and dangerous", despite its successful use in treating rheumatic diseases for decades.

Research in the last few years has vindicated the use of the galvanic bath, but in the most invasive way: Researchers are using implanted "electroceuticals" to stimulate the vagus nerve with a small current and inhibit the release of inflammatory-causing cytokines. Based on the former success of the Schnee bath, investigators were looking for a more modern medical way to treat autoimmune diseases like arthritis—but one that is more expensive and that they can control. SetPoint Medical Corporation has patented the device, called the *MicroRegulator*.

But naturopathic doctors can still produce the same results without resorting to surgical means, and with far less expense to the patient.

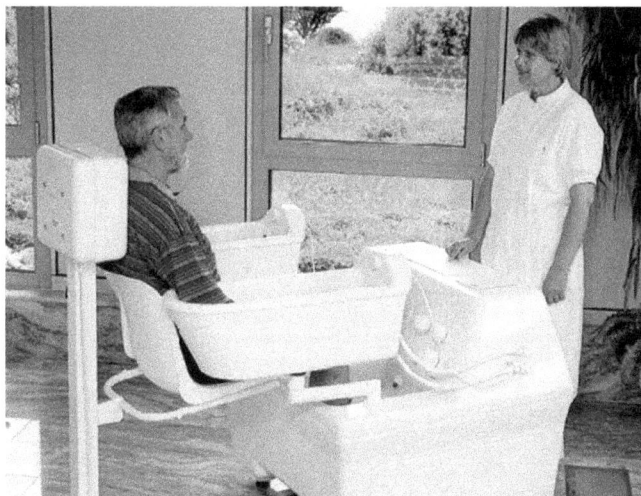

Above: Patient receiving treatment in Germany with **Trautwein** four cell apparatus, which is microprocessor controlled to deliver alternating temperatures in its cells as well.

Right: Four-cell apparatus manufactured by **Fizyomed®** of Turkey.

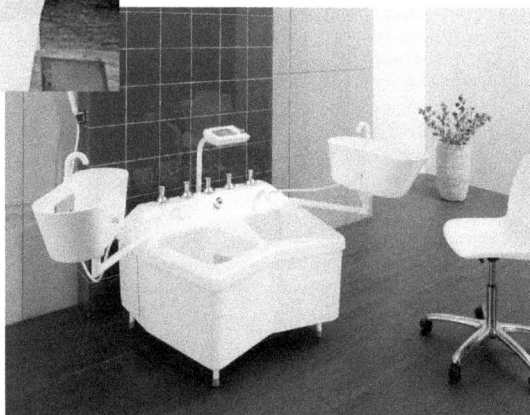

[3] Galvanic current is explained in detail in Chapter 6.

HYDROTHERAPY

CONSTITUTIONAL HYDROTHERAPY

H

DESCRIPTION
A unique and powerful form of hydrotherapy in which hot and cold compresses are applied to the torso, combined with electrical stimulation over several nerve centers with sine wave current.

EQUIPMENT NEEDED
- Treatment table
- Source of hot and cold water
- Containers large enough to soak towels in the hot and cold water
- 5 Terry cloth towels
- 2 blankets
- Oral thermometer
- Timer
- Urine specimen cup
- Urinalysis reagent strips
- Stethoscope
- **Sine wave** electrotherapy machine

EFFECTS AND PURPOSE
- Aside from the same effects from other types of alternating or contrast hydrotherapy (see **Alternating Bath**), constitutional hydrotherapy causes a very large amount of water to be absorbed into the body during the cold phase, which accounts for its powerful impact on accumulated toxic waste in the tissues.

INDICATIONS FOR USE
Practically any condition that will benefit from a boost in immune response and nutritional uptake by the tissues.
- Infections
- Hypersensitivity to environmental elements

- Gastrointestinal dysfunction
- Chronic respiratory conditions
- Hypertension
- Poor circulation
- Lymphatic congestion
- Dysmenorrhea
- Infertility
- Arthritis
- Hemorrhoids
- Varicose veins
- Immune deficiency

CONTRAINDICATIONS
- Acute asthma episode
- Acute bladder infection
- Malignant fever
- Standard contraindications for sine wave applications (i.e., pacemaker, over gravid uterus, etc.)

PRECAUTIONS
- Do not perform if the patient's urine specific gravity is below 1.015
- Do not perform if patient's oral temperature is below 97ºF. Warm the patient first.

ADVANTAGES
- So powerful and versatile that, if mastered, it makes many other hydrotherapy methods detailed in this book unnecessary.
- Shorter duration treatment times than other methods.

DISADVANTAGES
- Complex enough that it is initially daunting to learn; however, in a short time the muscle memory is gained from performing it so that it is no longer laborious.
- Since it combines electrotherapy with hydrotherapy, extra equipment is needed compared to other hydriatic procedures.

INSTRUCTIONS
1. Collect urine specimen from patient and measure specific gravity.
2. Place two woolen blankets on table.
3. Place sheet over blankets.
4. Patient undresses from waist up, puts on cloth gown or drape.
5. Place sine pads between shoulder blades at T5 level.
6. Insert towel at waistband to protect clothing.

7. Record patient's temperature.
8. Have patient lie on his/her back on the sheet.
9. Prepare two hot towels, wring out and place over chest and abdomen (each towel folded in half, making four layers total). Check temperature first with your wrist to ensure it will not burn patient.
10. Wrap patient in blankets. Leave in place and set timer for 5 minutes.
11. Prepare one hot and one cold towel and wring out.
12. At the five-minute mark, apply new hot towel on top of old hot towels and flip so that new hot towel is directly on patient.
13. Remove two old hot towels, leaving the one in contact with patient.
14. Immediately apply cold towel on top of hot towel and flip towels so that cold towel is against patient. Cover patient with blanket again.
15. Apply sine surge gradually to patient tolerance; leave this and cold towel on for 10 minutes <u>or until towel is fully warmed by the body</u>. Set timer for 10 minutes.
16. At ten-minute mark, turn off sine wave and check towel for warmth.
17. Remove towel and move one sine pad to L5, the other to solar plexus (or other abdominal location, depending on patient's needs). Restart surge to patient tolerance, or until you feel abdominal muscle contractions. Cover the patient with blanket and leave sine wave on for 10 minutes.
18. Remove pads, turn patient to prone position.
19. Place two hot towels on back.
20. Set timer for 5 minutes.
21. Repeat steps 10,11, and 12 while patient lies prone.
22. Set timer and leave cold towel on for 10 minutes, or until towel has warmed.
23. Remove towel and lightly dry patient's back.
24. Retake temperature and specific gravity and record in the chart.
25. Have the patient rest for a short time.
    <u>Important</u>: Never remove cold towel before it is warmed, or treatment may be ineffectual.

VARIATIONS:
- If oral temperature < 97° F, warm the patient before starting treatment.
- If oral temperature 97-98° F use an extra pair hot towels during hot towel phases; leave first pair of towels on for 4 minutes and apply second pair for 2 minutes.
- If oral temperature 99-100° F shorten hot towel phases from 5 to 3 minutes.
- If oral temperature 100-101° F shorten hot towel phases to 2 minutes and lengthen cold phases to 15 minutes.
- If oral temperature > 101° F shorten hot towel phases to 1 minute and lengthen cold phases to 15-20 minutes.
- If patient complains of feeling chilly use variation #2.
- If lung congestion is present use variation #2.
- If rheumatic condition, use variation #2.

- If extreme peripheral pain, apply hot compress to area during first hot towel phase.
- If congestion anywhere apply heat to feet, especially during cold phases
- If chronic pelvic problem, (ovaries, prostate, bladder) either:
- ·Apply 5 minutes of high frequency or short wave diathermy over the affected area instead of sine pad-only phase, or:
- Give standard treatment then end with 5 minutes of high frequency or short wave diathermy over affected area.
- If during healing crisis without fever adjust changes as follows: 5 min. hot to back, 10 min. cold to back, 10 min. intrascapular sine wave at T5, 10 min. sine to abdomen and L5, 5 min. hot to chest, 10 min. cold to chest
- If patient is tense and anxious use #12 variation above.
- For localized problems (i.e. fractures, diabetic ulcers, etc.) use an extra phase of continuous sine wave adjusted to only slightly perceptible intensity. Place one pad distal to affected area and the other pad over the spinal level governing innervation to affected area. Apply this before flipping patient over to prone position.

IN TREATING CHILDREN:
- Double the length of cold and hot phases
- No intrascapular sine pads
- No hot towels before changing to cold towels

FREQUENCY OF TREATMENT
As appropriate for the case.

REFERENCES
- Dick-Kronenberg, L., *The Ultimate Text In Constitutional Hydrotherapy*; 2014 Lulu
- Boyle, W., and Saine, A., *Lectures in Naturopathic Hydrotherapy*, Buckeye Naturopathic Press 1988

5

PHOTOTHERAPY

SUNLIGHT (Heliotherapy)

P

DESCRIPTION

Heliotherapy is the therapeutic use of the sun's rays. Its application involves a number of factors: latitude, altitude, climate, and clearness of air. As a therapeutic modality, it is always coupled with hygiene, diet, exercise, and rest. Naturally, the sun's rays contain the **infrared** rays and the **ultraviolet** rays, but the full extent of the life-giving properties of the sun are yet to be fully known. While this is a fundamental naturopathic modality, it was adopted by mainstream medicine and was once prevalent. It was a major modality in the treatment of tuberculosis in the pre-antibiotic era. At right we see the famous Dr. Rollier in his clinic in the Swiss Alps with tubercular patients. Hospitals of any size always had outdoor sun decks or indoor solariums, and could still be seen into the 1960s. Polio and arthritis patients alike were prescribed "sun time" every day.

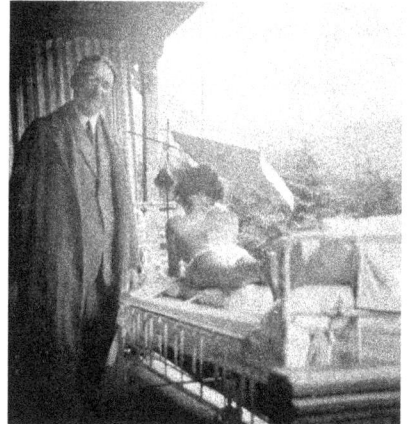

EQUIPMENT NEEDED
Sunlight.

It should be noted that "artificial sunlight" has been generated and used therapeutically with much success over the years; although realistically no device can fully reproduce *all* the factors present in sunlight. The lamps that have been used clinically, made by companies like Hanovia and Gilbert, have generated a wide sampling of the **ultraviolet**

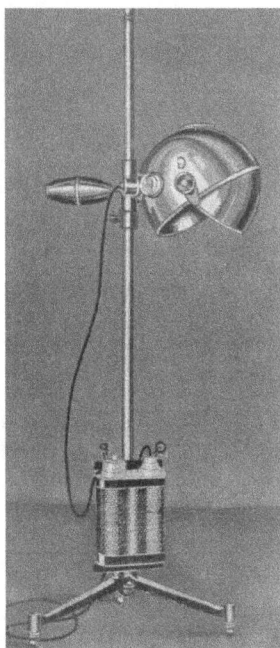

Alpine sun lamp
made by Hanovia

spectrum and a little **infrared**. While direct sunlight outdoors has been a mainstay of naturopathic resorts and sanitoriums (such as Benedict Lust's Yungborn Retreat), most clinical facilities in cities used some type of artificial sunlight as a therapy. Since this is mostly synonymous with **ultraviolet**, the specifics are covered in that chapter.

EFFECTS AND PURPOSE

Heliotherapy has a long history of improving appetite and sleep quality. It brings tone to both flabby flesh and muscle, so important to cases under bed rest or immobilization. The sinews regain tone and the sun's rays expand the subcutaneous tissue so that the flesh fills out. The sedimentation rate of the blood cells increases, Vitamin D is activated, and immune response is heightened. It should be noted that heliotherapy as practiced in mountain resorts contains one more element: aerotherapy. The mountain air plays a role in the effects of treatment, and some institutions would begin with exposure to the air only, covering the patient and gradually exposing different parts of the body. Cool air mixed with strong sun has a powerful tonic effect systemically.

INDICATIONS FOR USE
- Most systemic conditions
- Fatigue
- Poor appetite
- Sluggish metabolism
- Insomnia
- Headache

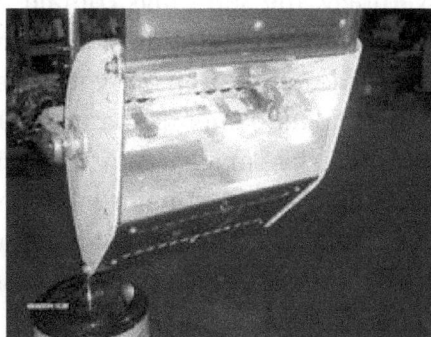

The author's own Hanovia Alpine lamp

CONTRAINDICATIONS
- Ulcerous enteritis with diarrhea
- Nephritis
- Amyloid degeneration
- Decompensated cardiac conditions

PRECAUTIONS
- Avoid overheating. This is especially critical when the sun is very hot and there is no wind.
- Scalp should be covered.
- Eyes should be protected from glare and ultraviolet rays.

ADVANTAGES

Does not require clinical setting.

DISADVANTAGES

Sunning has long been a recreational or cosmetic pastime and is not likely to be regarded seriously as a medical modality unless educated as to its use and effects.

INSTRUCTIONS

1. The best hours for exposure is when the air is clear and the heat is moderate. At a high elevation (mountains) in the summer, 7 AM to 11 AM and in the winter 10 AM to 3 PM.
2. Position can be prone or supine, or alternating.
3. Different parts of the body will have different degrees of sensitivity depending on the density of tissue.
4. Begin with suberythemal doses, first to a small portion of the body and gradually exposing more and more skin, as well as lengthening the time of exposure, always staying away from "sunburn" doses.
5. Eyes should always be protected with UV blocking glasses. The scalp should be covered.
6. On Day One, cover the body with a sheet or blanket and bare the feet for 5 minutes.
7. On Day Two, treat the feet for 10 minutes and expose the legs for the last five of those minutes by pulling the sheet up.
8. On Day Three, the thighs are added for the last 5 minutes (in addition to 10 minutes for the legs and 15 minutes for the feet).
9. On Day Four, the lower abdomen and loins are added for 5 minutes while the thighs get 10, the legs 15, and the feet 20 minutes.
10. On Day Five the entire front of the body is irradiated, with the thorax being added for 5 minutes.
11. On Day Six, the entire back is exposed for 5 minutes. There is no need at this point to segmentally expose the body.
12. Gradually increase exposure time each day. Always guard against overheating.
13. Exposure of 2-3 hours in summer and 3-4 hours in winter are possible once tanned.

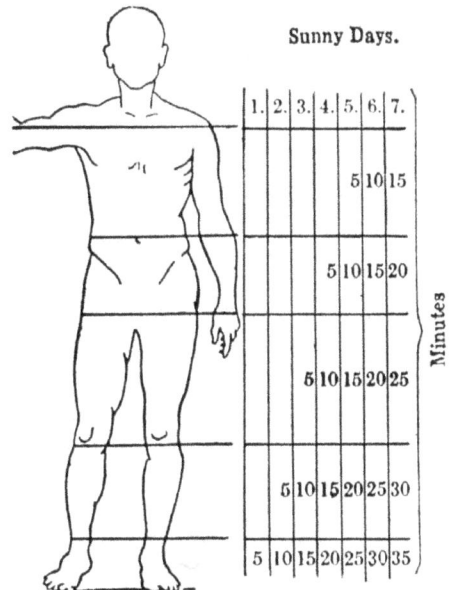

Rollier's guide, after Krusen

103

FREQUENCY OF TREATMENT
Already explained.

REFERENCES
- Michlovitz, S., *Thermal Agents in Rehabilitation*, 3rd Ed.; 1996 F.A. Davis Co. Lehmann, et.al., *Therapeutic Heat and Cold*; Ed.3, 1982 Williams & Wilkins
- Kovacs, R., *Light Therapy*; 1950 Charles C. Thomas
- Johnson, A.C., *Principles and Practice of Drugless Therapeutics*; 3rd Ed., 1946 Chiropractic Educational Extension Bureau
- Kellogg, J.H., *Light Therapeutics*; 1927 Modern medicine Pub. Co.

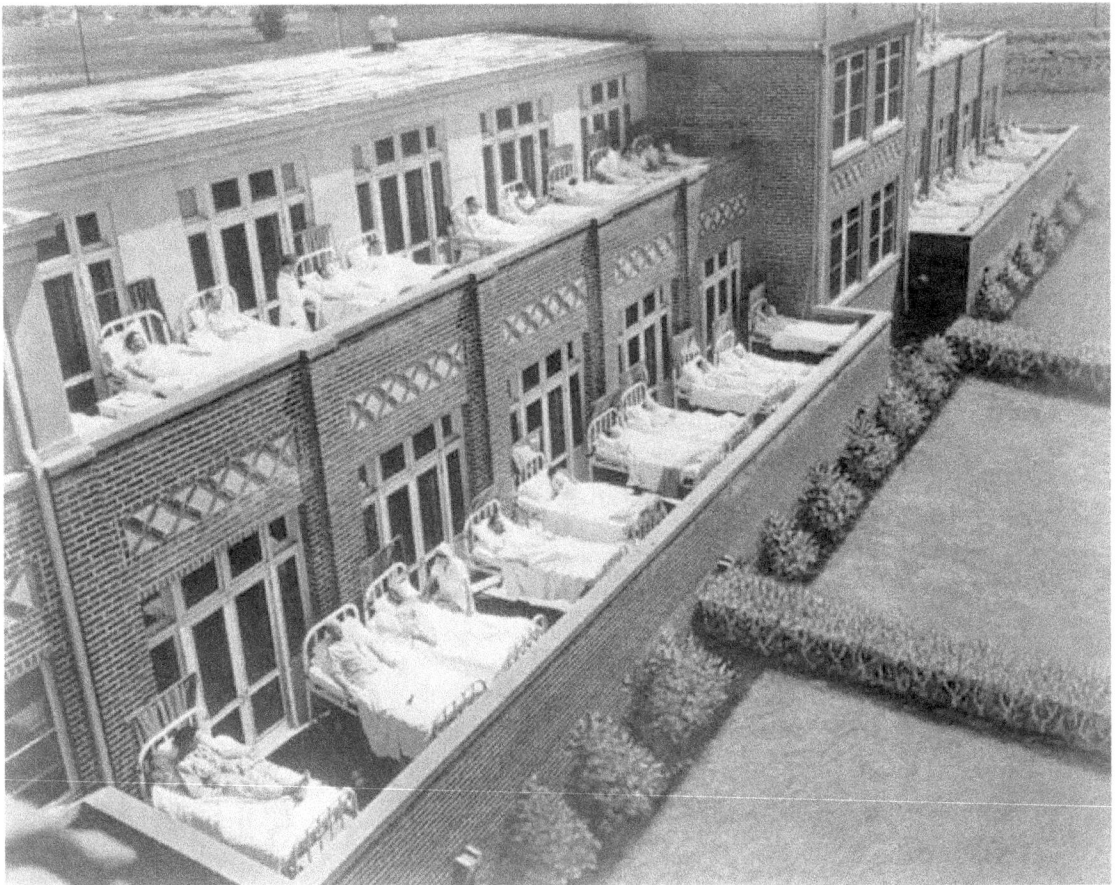

Institutional Heliotherapy

PHOTOTHERAPY

ELECTRIC LIGHT BATH

P

DESCRIPTION

The electric light cabinet is a piece of physiotherapeutic equipment no longer manufactured but included here because such a cabinet can still be constructed for little cost and may be desirable for a naturopathic clinic.

The Electric Light "Bath" is a treatment that straddles two categories, for though it uses light, it is also a delivery of radiant heat and therefore has a place in the **Thermotherapy** category. We have placed in in the **Light** section here.

The cabinet is generally an upright one (although reclining ones have been made), similar to a **Russian Bath** or **Finnish Bath** but the heating element is the incandescent light. Incandescents produce not only luminous visible light but also quantities of infrared (which is why a light bulb becomes hot). The cabinet is wood or metal and contains a number of (usually) 80 Watt light bulbs[4] arranged on the inner sides. The wiring is designed so that banks of lights can be turned on or off, thus regulating the heat. The cabinet is partially open at the top and has an air vent in the center bottom.

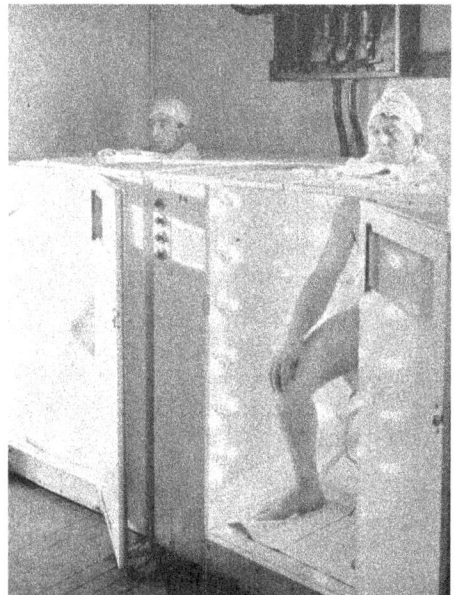

---

[4] Near infrared bulbs would be the preferred filaments used today, with the decline of incandescent bulbs.

EQUIPMENT NEEDED
- Light cabinet or some enclosed space with the appropriate light/heat elements
- Towel
- Cold soaked towel for head wrap
- Oral thermometer
- Lukewarm water for the patient to sip

EFFECTS AND PURPOSE
Luminous (visible light) heat causes an erythema within a few minutes. The skin becomes hot and red by means of the vasomotor mechanism and dilates the capillaries, leading to a secondary increase in arterial and venous circulation. The infrared rays, which penetrate more deeply, activate the sweat glands in subcutaneous tissue, leading to perspiration within a short time. Since large areas of the skin are exposed in an electric light bath, the effect is global. The results are:

- Increased heat elimination and perspiration
- Increased circulation
- Induction of therapeutic fever
- Raised pulse rate (10 bpm for each degree of temperature raised)
- Lowering of blood pressure
- Increased respiration
- Increased elimination through the kidneys

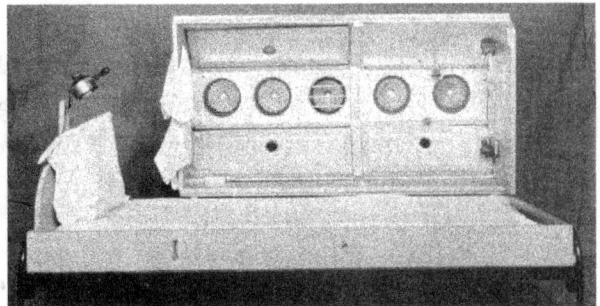

A reclining luminous cabinet

INDICATIONS FOR USE
- General toxicity
- Infection (for which fever induction is indicated)
- Subacute or chronic inflammation
- Arthritis and other rheumatic conditions
- Neuritis, boils and carbuncles
- Aid in systemic detoxification
- Aid to athletic recovery
- Aid to peripheral circulation

CONTRAINDICATIONS
- Open wounds
- Dermatitis

- Swelling or bruising at site
- Multiple sclerosis patients
- Diabetic patients
- Patients with deep vein thrombosis (DVTs)
- Patients with other vascular diseases (the risk of burn if the circulation is not adequate to dissipate heat in the tissues)

PRECAUTIONS
- Patients with neurosensory problems cannot judge the level of heat, requiring careful monitoring of such patients. The same goes for patients with confusion.
- Existing edema can be aggravated by radiant heat.   Mild intensity should be used, along with elevation.

ADVANTAGES
- Disrobing is not as much an issue when the body is concealed in a cabinet

DISADVANTAGES
- Operator must monitor patient's condition and temperature
- Patient must be cautious about staying away from the bulbs
- Repeated long exposure can lead to permanent mottled pigmentation, like the veins in marble

INSTRUCTIONS
1. Turn on lights in the cabinet in advance to warm the inside air.
2. Patient is cautioned about avoiding the heat sources inside the cabinet.
3. Conduct the patient, wrapped in a sheet or gown, to the cabinet.
4. The covering is removed as the patient sits on a low stool.
5. The cabinet lid is closed, leaving the patient's head exposed.
6. The head is covered with a cold moist compress.
7. Patient may drink tepid water freely during the bath through a straw and is encouraged to, in order to assist elimination.
8. Operator should remain with the patient.
9. If patient feels faint or the pulse rises above 100 bpm, the procedure should be terminated.
10. The duration should be a brief 5-8 minutes if tonic action is desired (typically the point of beginning perspiration).
11. The duration should be 8-15 minutes if detoxification is the desired result.

It is a rule that the patient must not leave the premises until thoroughly cooled off. In facilities that are equipped, the patient should take a brief cool shower after; it is optimal to have a **Scotch douche** if possible.

FREQUENCY OF TREATMENT

For tonic purposes, daily or every other day.   For elimination/detoxification, twice weekly.

REFERENCES

- Kovacs, R., *Light Therapy;* 1950 Charles C. Thomas
- Kovacs, R., *Electrotherapy and Light Therapy;* 6th Ed., 1949 Lea & Febiger
- Johnson, A.C., *Principles and Practice of Drugless Therapeutics;* 3rd Ed., 1946 Chiropractic Educational Extension Bureau
- Krusen, F., *Physical Medicine;* 1941 W. B. Saunders Co.
- Mayer, E., *Clinical Application of Sunlight and Artificial Radiation;* 1925 Williams & Wilkins

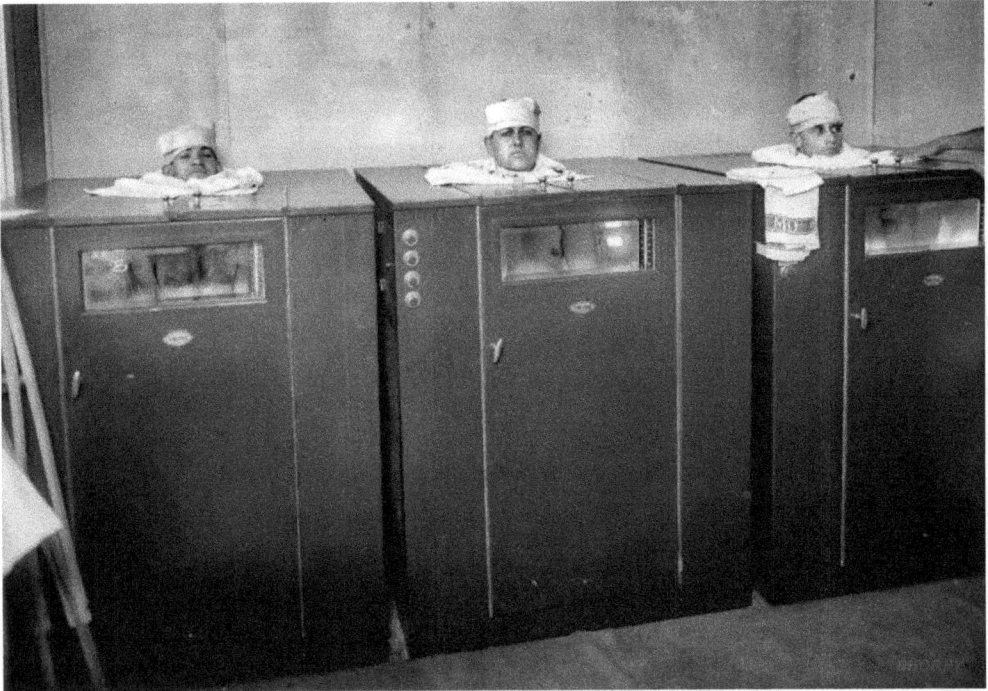

Military men being treated at Walter Reed Hospital

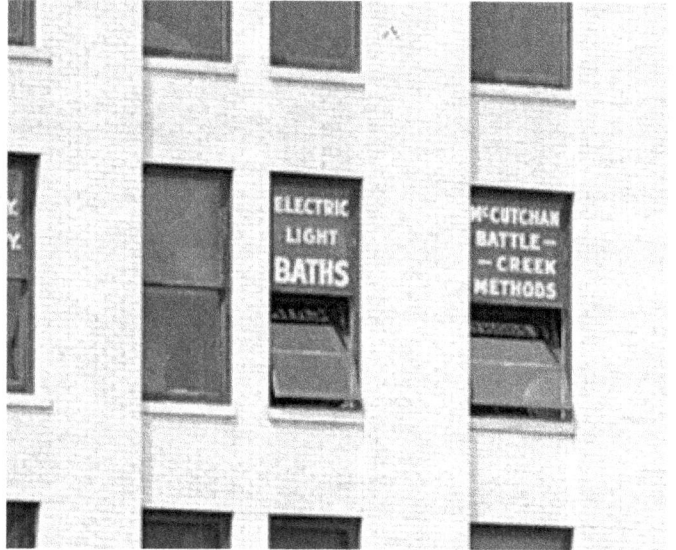

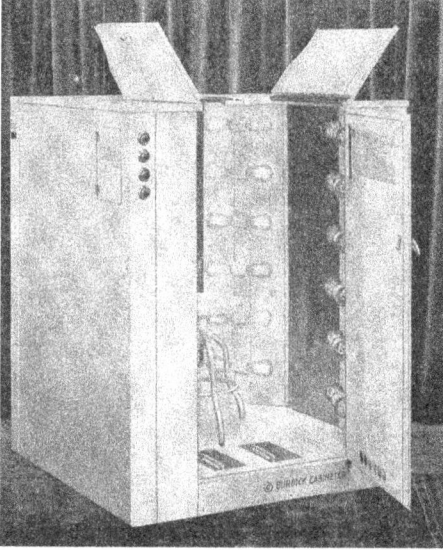

Burdick Corporation, although they today make only medical equipment like electrocardiographs, was a major manufacturer of physiotherapeutic devices used by naturopathic doctors for decades. They even had their version of the electric light cabinet.

Naturopathic clinic in the Keenan Building, downtown Pittsburgh Pennsylvania. Electric light baths were far from an obscure therapy.

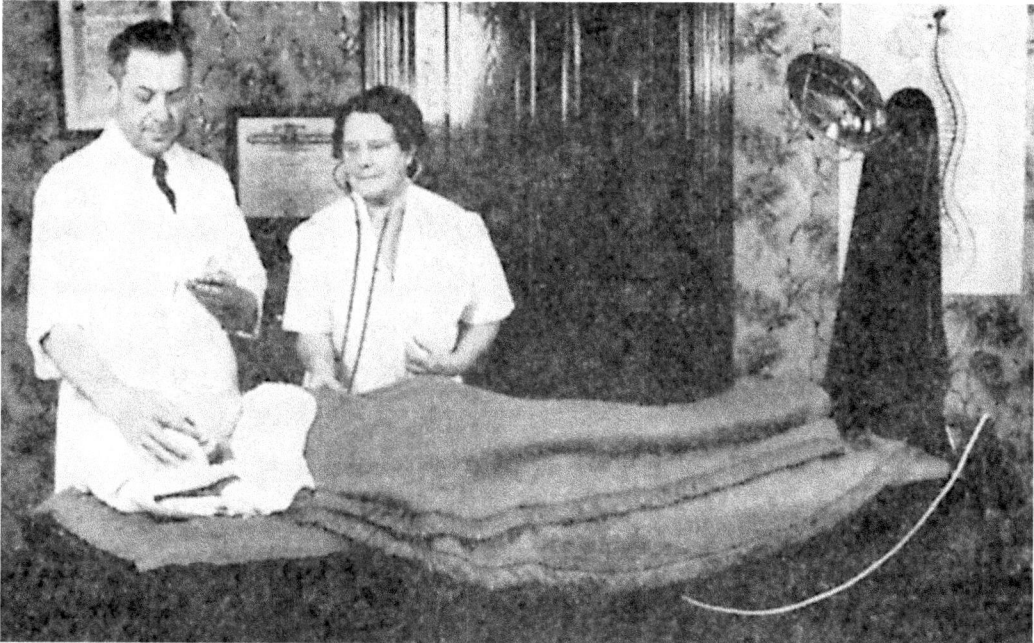

Chloe Jay, ND monitors a patient undergoing hyperpyrexia (fever) treatment in an enclosure filled with hot air instead of heat lamps, ca. 1940. Note the fan to cool the patient's head.

110

PHOTOTHERAPY

CHROMOTHERAPY

P

DESCRIPTION

Chromotherapy, as the name implies, is treatment with colored light. The frequencies in the visible light spectrum have therapeutic effects, just as those in the invisible parts of the spectrum (infrared, ultraviolet, etc.)

EQUIPMENT NEEDED

After vicious persecution decades ago, color projectors for medical use have generally not been manufactured since. Home users and practitioners have constructed their own and suffered no loss of efficacy as a result. The more important matter is the correct color filters to produce the correct frequencies of light. There are several producers of these, as color gels are used for stage and movie lighting and cannot be outlawed. Basically any light source with a structure that will hold a color filter, and channel the light through that filter, will work.

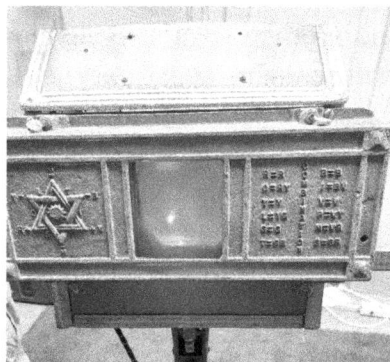

Original Dinshah color projector

The recommended source for color filters is Rosco Laboratories (www.us.rosco.com), who make gels that create the accurate frequencies of light for each of the colors, as determined by decades of research. You will notice that the correct shade is produced most of the time by combining two or three filters, as seen in this Roscolene filter list at right.

Further advice on setting up chromotherapy equipment can be had from Dinshah Health Society at https://dinshahhealth.org.

Roscolene Filter Combinations
Red = R818, R828
Yellow = R809
Green = R871
Blue = R859, R866
Violet = R832, R859, R866
Magenta = R818, R828, R866
Orange = R809, R828
Lemon = R809, R871
Turquoise = R861, R871
Indigo = R828, R859, R866

EFFECTS AND PURPOSE

Every element, when placed in a spectroscope, gives off a distinctive identifying set of emission lines, color bands (called Fraunhofer lines) that are specific to that substance. When exposed to light, the element will absorb from the light those frequencies (colors) that they characteristically give off. Therefore, full-spectrum white light (which contains all colors) acts as a "nutrient" for the element. Limiting the light to only that color intensifies the absorption of the characteristic color.

Pioneering researchers Dinshah and Loeb each matched the Fraunhofer lines associated with a particular element to find the color related to its function. Then sick people's conditions that were associated with a dysfunction of that element in the body were treated with that color, and observed for changes. This has led to a large repository of knowledge regarding which colors have been found to act positively on which illnesses[5].

As a general theory it is accepted that in disease, the structural patterns of the neural pathways are abnormally aligned. Chromotherapy appears to release chemicals that accomplish a re-alignment of those pathways with enhanced nerve cell growth. On a more broad level, mal-illumination (a condition resulting from missing frequencies of natural light, due to artificial lighting or insufficient exposure to sunlight) can be a causative factor in disease, and corrected by supplying exposure to the colors the person is lacking.

Dinshah's theory was that since spectroscopy proves that each element emanated its own specific frequency of light, a sort of "vibrational fingerprint", that illness produced changes in those frequencies in different tissues. Disharmony between the various systems in the body with their composite frequencies would be a disease state, which could then be manipulated with the needed frequencies of light (colors) that would return resonance to the abnormal, out-of-phase state at the molecular level. Matter being simply condensed light, as it is now referred to in modern physics, it follows that action on matter by use of colored light is not such a metaphysical proposition as formerly thought. At any rate, many decades of successful use with thousands of case histories on record confirm chromotherapy's place in the naturopathic armamentarium.

---

[5] Naturopath Harry Riley Spitler did the same, but concentrated on application through the eyes to create neurological changes via the brain. Spitler theorized that the stimulation of either the sympathetic or parasympathetic nerves by the colored light was the mechanism by which his chromotherapy worked, since illness was seen to be a disequilibrium of the autonomic nervous system. Today, it is well established that visual stimulation creates the "entrainment" response in the brain, and habitual patterns can be offset by application of interrupted bursts of color along the optic nerve, thus interrupting those patterns and helping establish new ones. For this reason, chromotherapy has been applied by Syntonic optometrists with great success in emotional problems and information processing disorders.

COLOR ATTRIBUTES AND USES

RED: Stimulates sensory nerves; sights, smell, taste, touch, and hearing. Tonic to the liver; Builds hemoglobin; Causes expulsion of debris through the skin; Causes erythema, itching, skin vesicles may appear until the healing process is complete.

ORANGE: Stimulates respiratory organs; Thyroid stimulant; Parathyroid depressant; Bone builder; Antispasmodic; Stimulates mammary glands to produce milk (galactagogue); Tonic to stomach and assists vomiting (emetic); Reduces gas and flatulence (carminative).

YELLOW: Stimulates motor nerves; Stimulates lymphatic system; Stimulates intestinal activity, production of digestive fluids; Stimulates the pancreas; Increases bowel movements (cathartic); Expels worms and parasites; Inhibits the spleen; Balances mood in depression.

LEMON: Stimulates nutritional uptakes and tissue repair in long term disorders (chronic alterative); Stimulates coughing if needed (expectorant); Assists bone growth by activating phosphorus; Stimulates the brain; Stimulates the thymus; Mild stimulant to the GI tract (mild laxative effect).

GREEN: Physical balancer; Stimulates pituitary; Stimulates re-building of muscles; Germicidal; Disinfectant; Antiseptic.

TURQUOISE: Accelerates nutritional uptake and tissue repair in recent disorders (acute alterative); Inhibits excess brain activity; Rebuilds burned skin (antipyrotic); Skin tonic.

BLUE: Relieves itching (anti-pruritic); Relieves irritation of abraded surfaces (demulcent); Induces perspiration (diaphoretic); Reduced fever (antipyretic) or inflammation (antiphlogistic); Stimulates pineal gland; Builds vitality.

INDIGO: Stimulates parathyroid; Inhibits thyroid; Respiratory depressant; Causes constriction that arrests hemorrhage (hemostatic) and discharges (astringent); Mammary depressant, reducing milk production; Increases production of phagocytes and the destruction of harmful microorganisms; Lessens excitement and hyperactivity (sedative).

VIOLET: Stimulates the spleen; Decreases muscle activity, including the heart (muscular and cardiac depressant); Lymphatic system depressant; Decreases activity of motor nerves; Promotes leukocyte production.

PURPLE: Kidney depressant; Raises pain threshold; Induces relaxation and sleep (soporific); Lowers blood pressure by vasodilation, reducing heart rate, and lowering activity of the chromaffin system; Lowers body temperature (antipyretic); Helps control fever and blood pressure in periodic diseases (antimalarial); Lowers sex drive when excessive (anaphrodisiac).

MAGENTA: Emotional balancer; Equilibrates activity of heart and vascular system, adrenals, and the chromaffin system.

SCARLET: Stimulates kidneys; Raises blood pressure by contraction of the blood vessels, increasing heart rates and stimulating the chromaffin system; Raises sex drive by increasing desire when deficient (aphrodisiac); Stimulates the menstrual function (emmenagogue); Accelerate expulsion of fetus st time of delivery (ecbolic).

INDICATIONS FOR USE
Virtually any condition

CONTRAINDICATIONS
Virtually none, although temporary exacerbation can occur if a
color inimical to the condition is used, or if it is applied too powerfully.

PRECAUTIONS
The light projector needs to be stable so that heat generated by the filament and transferred to the housing does not accidentally burn the patient.

ADVANTAGES
- "Low tech" simplicity
- Little manual skill needed for procedure
- Can be used at home competently by patient as well

DISADVANTAGES
- Typically long treatment time
- Need for darkening the treatment room for best results

INSTRUCTIONS
1. Select appropriate color slide and insert into the projector.
2. Position patient with the area to be treated exposed.
3. Darken room and turn on projector.
4. Allow the target area to be bathed in the colored light for the determined length of time

FREQUENCY OF TREATMENT

Typical Dinshah-style treatment recommends an hour's exposure ("tonation") daily.

REFERENCES

- DInshah, D., *Let There Be Light;* 13th Ed., 2021 Dinshah Health Society
- Dinshah, D., *Spectro-Chrome Guide: Abridged Manual for Spectro-Chrome Therapy;* 1997 Dinshah Health Society
- Anderson. M., *Colour Healing: Chromotherapy and How It Works;* 1975 Samuel Weiser Co.
- Douglas, W., *Into the Light;* 1993 Second Opinion Publishing Johnson,
- Lieberman, J., *Light, Medicine of the Future;* 1991 Bear & Co.
- A.C., *Principles and Practice of Drugless Therapeutics;* 3rd Ed., Chiropractic Educational Extension Bureau 1946

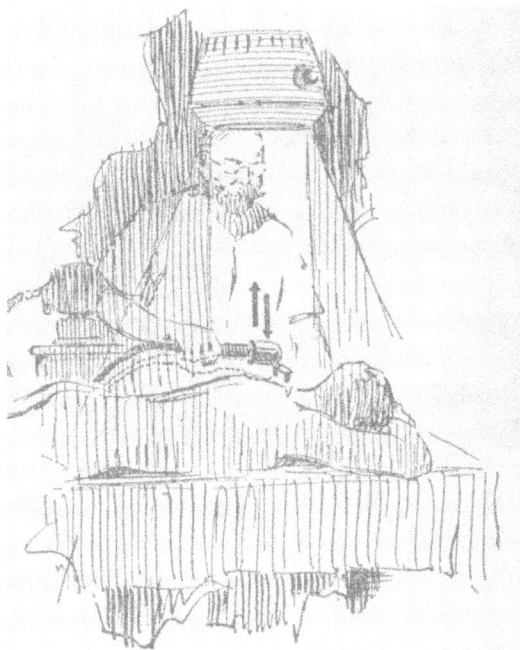

Chromotherapy combines well with other physiotherapies.

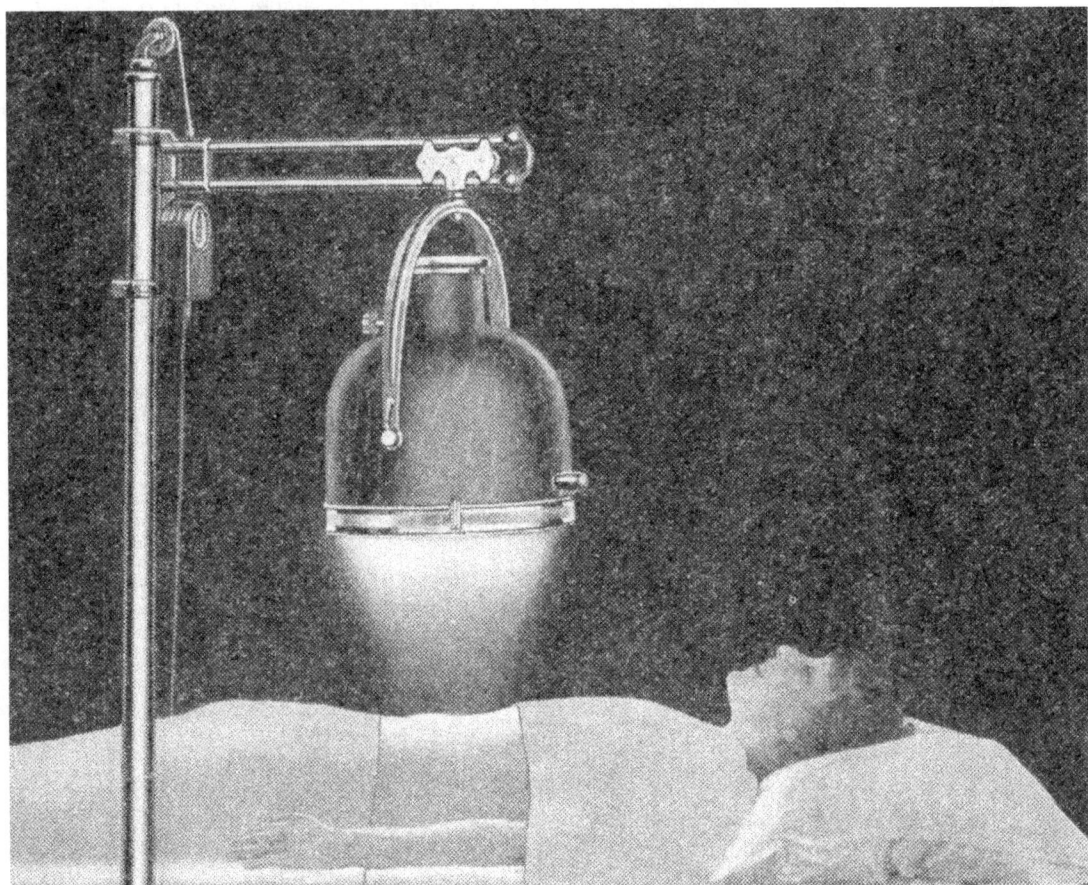

PHOTOTHERAPY

INFRARED

P

DESCRIPTION

Infrared has been described in Chapter 2 on **radiant heat**.

As a type of convective heat, infrared operates on a simple physical principle. It activates vasomotor reflexes that direct a greater volume of blood to be rushed to the part treated, simultaneously stimulating the expelling of as much of the excess heat as possible in an instinctive defense against tissue damage. The result is the reflex action can also take an action on adjacent and even distant parts of the body. Therefore, a more systemic response of increased blood flow and excretion of waste products in the tissues is created.

It is important to note that increasing the degree of heat applied will not cause a deeper penetration and affect underlying tissues, for the very reason explained above.

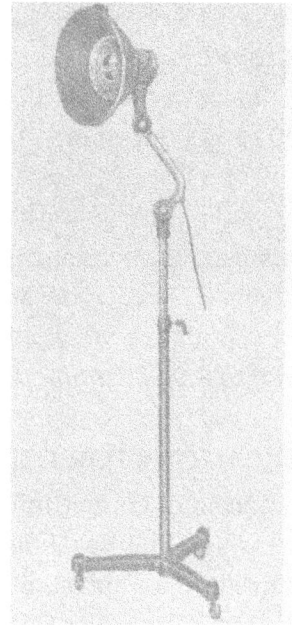

EQUIPMENT NEEDED

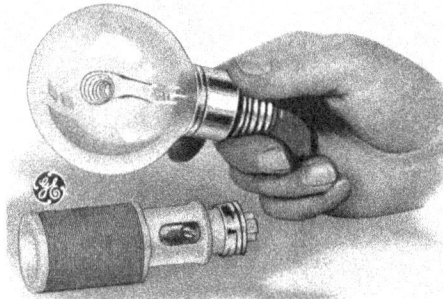

A radiant heat lamp, either luminous or non-luminous. Luminous bulbs are usually tungsten filament bulbs and produce mainly short wave (near) infrared waves. Non-luminous lamps are typically a carborundum core with a reflector, and produce mainly long wave (far) infrared waves.
A comparison of these (courtesy of General Electric) can be seen here.

117

Carbon arc lamps were one type of radiant heat used in Naturopathy in times past. This type of equipment was superseded over time and replaced by infrared lamps, and then the carbon arc lamps ceased being manufactured. They are mentioned for completeness.

EFFECTS AND PURPOSE

Long wave (far) infrared is absorbed in the stratum corneum of the epidermis, only 1-2 mm. Yet, it is known to reduce pain, accelerate skin healing, lower blood pressure, increase peripheral circulation, benefit chronic kidney disease, and modulate autoimmune responses. Its use in full-body saunas is well known today. The filaments are in the frequency range of 2000 to 3,000 nanometers.

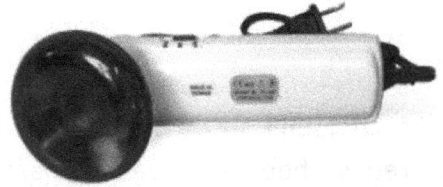

Infralux, a small hand-held device is easy to use and affordable.

Short wave (near) infrared penetrates deeply, 5-10 mm, affecting vascular beds in the dermis and nerve endings. The waves affect arterial and venous circulation and they stimulate more perspiration than long wave infrared. They stimulate energy production in the mitochondria. They are in the frequency range of 780 to 3,000 nanometers.

INDICATIONS FOR USE
• Subacute or chronic inflammation
• Arthritis and other rheumatic conditions
• Neuritis, boils and carbuncles
• Aid in systemic detoxification
• Aid to athletic recovery
• Aid to peripheral circulation

CONTRAINDICATIONS
• Open wounds
• Dermatitis
• Swelling or bruising at site
• Multiple sclerosis patients
• Diabetic patients
• Patients with deep vein thrombosis (DVTs)
• Patients with other vascular diseases

PRECAUTIONS
- Patients with neurosensory problems cannot judge the level of heat, requiring careful monitoring of such patients. The same goes for patients with confusion.
- Existing edema can be aggravated by radiant heat. Mild intensity should be used, along with elevation.

ADVANTAGES
- No contact is made with the device, so no tenderness or balking at touch.
- The non-contact eliminates the contamination of wounds.
- The part treated can be continually monitored.

DISADVANTAGES
- Radiant heat cannot be used if the patient cannot be positioned properly to expose the target area.
- A small target area is difficult to irradiate due to the spread of the waves from the device to the body (although this can be remedied by a shroud made of cardboard with a hole the appropriate size cut into it) .

INSTRUCTIONS
1. Always check equipment first.
2. Non-luminous lamps should be turned on 5-10 minutes before application.
3. Explain the procedure to the patient. Have patient remove all jewelry and clothing from the area to be treated.
4. Drape the patient for modesty, but expose the area to be treated. Position the patient so that the target area for treatment is accessible.
5. Check patient's ability to sense heat and inspect skin for lesions that may preclude treatment.
6. Position the lamp in such way that a majority of the waves will hit the body at a right angle (perpendicular).
7. Measure the distance from the filament to the skin and record it in your notes.
8. Tell the patient that a comfortable warmth is the goal and not the limit that the patient can stand. Emphasize that patient should not move closer to the lamp or touch it. If unable to have constant monitoring, give patient a bell or other alarm to summon help if uncomfortable.
9. Treat for 15-20 minutes; a chronic condition needs 20-30 minutes.
10. Turn off and remove lamp. Dry the patient's skin and cover. Allow patient to rest for a few minutes before rising.

Note: The patient may adapt to the heat level after a time and request a higher intensity. *Moving the lamp closer risks burning the patient* because of the inability to judge it accurately.

Remember that the source-to-skin distance is what determines the amount of heat. A non-luminous lamp (carborundum core) producing far infrared with a 750 to 1000 watt output should be placed 36 inches away, measured from skin to the filament, raising or lowering later as needed.

A luminous lamp of 1000 watts should be placed at 30 inches to start. Smaller bulbs (500-600 watts) can be placed at 24 inches, and all can be raised or lowered as needed.

FREQUENCY OF TREATMENT
Daily, or even twice daily in subacute conditions. Chronic conditions should be treated once or twice a week.

REFERENCES
- Michlovitz, S., *Thermal Agents in Rehabilitation,* 3rd Ed.; 1996 F.A. Davis Co.
- Lehmann, et.al., *Therapeutic Heat and Cold*; Ed.3, 1982 Williams & Wilkins
- Kovacs, R., *Light Therapy*; 1950 Charles C. Thomas
- Johnson, A.C., *Principles and Practice of Drugless Therapeutics*; 3rd Ed., Chiropractic Educational Extension Bureau 1946
- Kellogg, J.H., *Light Therapeutics;* 1927 Modern medicine Pub. Co.

PHOTOTHERAPY

ULTRAVIOLET

P

DESCRIPTION

Ultraviolet light is in the wavelength band of 100-400 nm (nanometers) and is divided into three bands of its own: UVA (320 – 400 nm), UVB (280 – 320 nm), and UVC (100 – 280 nm).

All three types are produced by the sun, but the waves shorter than 290 nm (UVC) are absorbed by the atmosphere and do not make it to the earth. Those shorter waves can be created by artificial means and are used therapeutically.

UV therapy can be given locally (for skin lesions, etc.), or full body for general or constitutional benefit.

EQUIPMENT NEEDED

Two types of apparatus have been commonly used.

1. High pressure, air-cooled mercury vapor quartz glass tubes are typical. An electric current is passed through the generator and it vaporizes the mercury, causing the bulb to emit all three UV bands. This has been discussed in the section on artificial sunlight in the **Heliotherapy** chapter.

2. Cold quartz generators function much like the hot quartz type, but only emit the UVC waves, and have typically been used for orificial treatment and acute care, being smaller and lightweight. It is also suited to being used at a close distance.

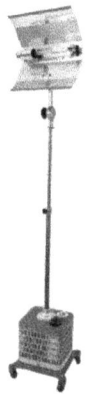

EFFECTS AND PURPOSE

• General tonic
• Increases resistance to infection (causes endothelial cells in the deep epidermis to produce more antibodies in the presence of bacteria)
• Direct germicidal action topically

- Lowers blood pressure
- Generates Vitamin D from 7-Dehydrocholesterol in the epidermis
- Increases calcium and phosphorus in the blood
- Increases volume of red blood cells, hemoglobin, and iron in the blood
- Stimulates thyroid gland and increases concentration of iodine in the blood
- Improves appetite, nutritional uptake, and sleep
- Locally, UV treatment releases a vasodilation substance in the epidermis that stimulates epithelial cell growth and promotes healing of wounds and skin lesions

INDICATIONS FOR USE
- Psoriasis
- Pruritus
- Slow healing wounds
- Acne vulgaris
- Arthritis

CONTRAINDICATIONS
- High fever
- Patients hypersensitive to the sun
- Acute pulmonary tuberculosis

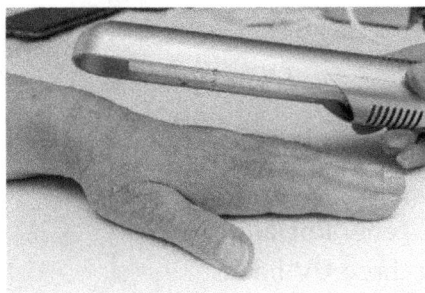
Psoriasis treatment

PRECAUTIONS
•Acute eczema and or dermatitis may be aggravated with localized exposure
•Systemic lupus erythematosus may be aggravated with localized exposure
•Hyperthyroid or diabetic patients may experience itching if given general exposure

ADVANTAGES
•Brief duration of therapy
•Conventionally accepted therapy

DISADVANTAGES
•Care must be taken so as not to overexpose the patient
•Equipment is used for a narrow range of conditions, but price has come down on the apparatus in recent years

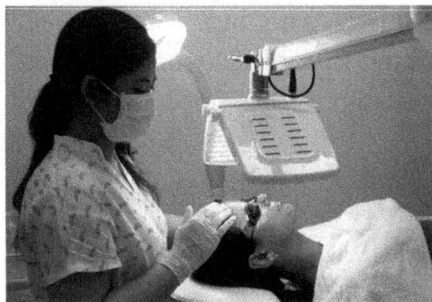
Acne treatment

PRE-THERAPY INSTRUCTIONS

Whether given in a small, local area, or given in a constitutional, tonic dose, the appropriate exposer time needs to be assessed first. The minimal erythemal dose (MED) is performed before initiating therapy.

1. Cut a test strip from paper or cloth (cotton or other fabric), 6 x 10 inches.
2. Cut holes in the various shapes as illustrated in the example.
3. Explain the procedure to the patient.
4. Choose an area of skin that is untanned, preferably one typically covered like the abdomen or chest. Wash and dry the area first. Remove all jewelry.
5. Drape patient appropriately to have only the test area exposed.
6. Attach the MED mask to the chosen area, making sure it lies flat against the skin.
7. Cover the mask with a towel.
8. Have a stopwatch ready.
9. Position the UV lamp directly over the area, parallel to the surface of the skin, 30 inches away from the highest point on the body.
10. Pull the towel back to expose the first hole in the mask, open the shutters of the generator to allow the UV light to shine on the target, and start the timer. Always step away from the lamp each time to avoid exposure yourself.
11. At the 30-second mark, expose the second hole also, by pulling the towel back farther. Expose for another 30 seconds.
12. Expose the third hole for 15 seconds.
13. Expose the fourth hole for 15 seconds.
14. Expose the fifth hole for 15 seconds.
15. Expose the sixth hole for 15 seconds.
16. Close shutters, turn lamp away from patient and shut it off.

The first hole will have been exposed for 120 seconds and the last one 15 seconds.
Ask the patient to check the area in a brightly lit room every two hours and report which shapes have appeared on the skin and at what time they fade. A form is included here to use for them to fill out and return on their next visit.

The minimal erythemal dose (MED) is the shortest dose to appear in 1-6 hours from the exposure and to disappear in 24 hours.

On the chance that all shapes remain visible after 24 hours, the test must be repeated with shorter dosage/exposure times.

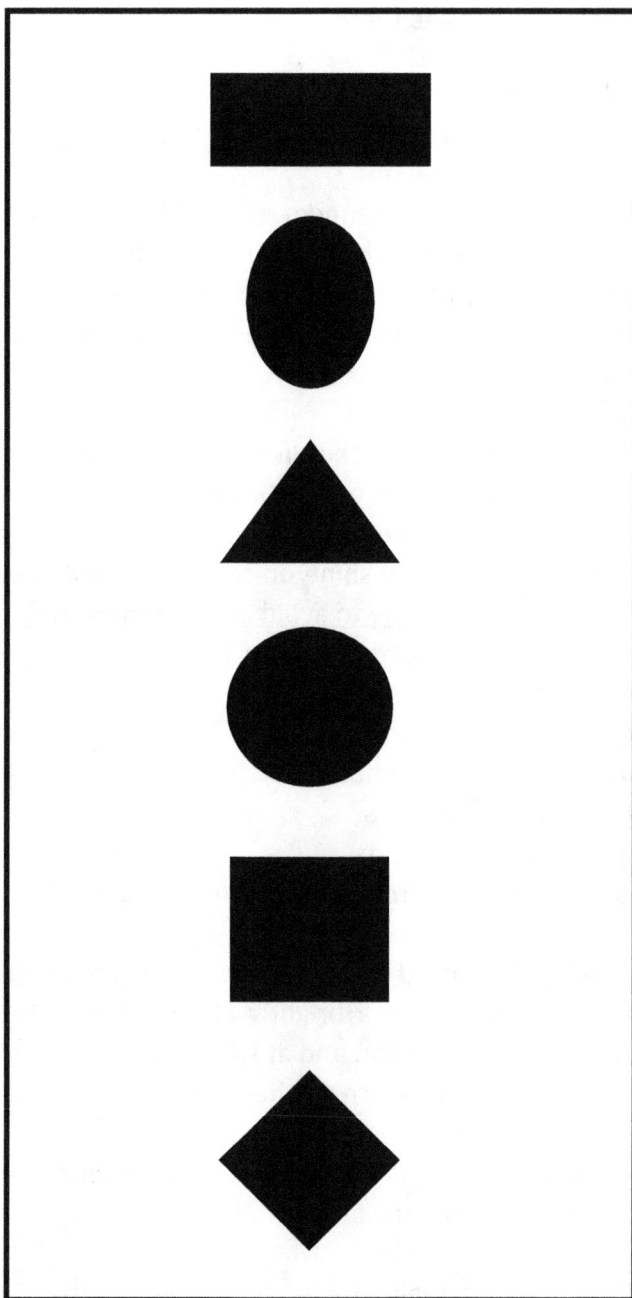

M.E.D. TEST FORM

Patient_____. Date_____

Site_____ Skin-lamp distance_____MED_____

# Hours	Shape					
	◆ 15	■ 30	● 45	▲ 60	⬭ 90	▬ 120
1						
2						
3						
4						
5						
6						
7						
8						
9						
10						
11						
12						
13						
14						
15						
16						
17						
18						
19						
20						
21						
22						
23						
24						

INSTRUCTIONS FOR GENERAL TREATMENT

1. Turn on machine to warm up filament for 3-5 minutes.
2. Give patient protective goggles and explain procedure.
3. Position nude patient in supine position, no pillow on table. Adjust goggles, place protective coverings over nipples and genitalia. Place arms in anatomical position and turn head to one side.
4. Drape patient completely with two sheets, one covering the lower half of the body, one covering the upper half. Edges should touch each other evenly and the sides should be tucked in to prevent moving.
5. Center the UV filament over the upper half of patient's body at the distance used for testing (typically 30 inches).
6. Remove upper sheet, without disturbing lower one.
7. Open UV shutters and expose for the length of time determined by the MED test.
8. Close shutters and replace the sheet in exactly the same position as before.
9. Move lamp over the lower body and re-check proper distance measurement.
10. Remove lower sheet.
11. Open shutters and deliver timed MED dose once again.
12. Turn patient prone, head to the opposite side as before (still with no pillow), and drape in the same manner as before.
13. Move lamp over the upper body again and re-check proper distance measurement.
14. Remove upper sheet, without disturbing lower one.
15. Open shutters and deliver timed MED dose again.
16. Close shutters and replace the sheet in exactly the same position as before.
17. Remove lower sheet.
18. Open shutters and deliver timed MED dose once again.
19. Replace the draping, remove the lamp, and allow patient to dress.

TYPICAL HOT QUARTZ EXPOSURE SCHEDULE

Tx #	Distance (inches)	Time
1	30	1
2	30	3
3	30	5
4	30	7
5	30	9
6	30	11
7	30	13
8	30	15
9	28	15
10	26	15
11	24	15
12	22	15

All doses are subject to modification, of course, based on the age and condition of the patient, the complexion, and the condition(s) treated.

If second degree erythema is produced, the sessions must be spaced more widely to avoid too many strong reactions in rapid succession.

INSTRUCTIONS FOR LOCALIZED TREATMENT

Localized treatment depends on whether a hot quartz or cold quartz lamp is being used. Hot quartz can be used for smaller areas, but draping must be done as in general treatment, so as to remove the rest of the body from exposure. Hot quartz should never be used at a distance of less than 15 inches, but can be used at closer range by using this formula:

$$\text{New time} = \text{initial time} \times \text{distance}_2 \div \text{new distance}$$

Cold quartz is designed to be used at shorter distances.

DOSE	DISTANCE (inches)	EXPOSURE (seconds)
MED	1	12-15
T_1	1	36-45
T_2	1	72-90
T_3	1	135-180

1. Turn on machine to warm up filament for 3-5 minutes if it requires warmup.
2. Give patient protective goggles and explain procedure.
3. Wash and dry area to be treated. Any topical medication should be removed.
4. Drape patient appropriately (use sterile drapes if a wound is present).
5. Position filament so that the UV waves will be perpendicular to the skin.
6. Create a stable one-inch distance from the filament to the skin.
7. Dosage is dependent on condition. Lesions or wounds in the process of healing can be treated with either the MED or T_1 dose (see below). Infected wounds or ulcerated tissue can be treated with T_2 or T_3 doses for germicidal action and to stimulate repair. If the MED cannot be determined, use the following guide:

FREQUENCY OF TREATMENT

Ultraviolet treatment should not be repeated until the effects of the previous exposure have vanished. Exposures should be increased by 25% with each new exposure to create the same level of response (except for mucosal tissue, which remains the same[6]). For each missed session, the following exposure should be <u>decreased</u> by 25%. If some time has elapsed without treatments, or if there has been skin peeling (desquamation), the dose should be returned to the original MED.

----

[6] Mucosal tissue has no epidermal covering.

REFERENCES

- Michlovitz, S., *Thermal Agents in Rehabilitation*, 3rd Ed.; 1996 F.A. Davis Co.
- Shriber, W.J., *Manual of Eletrcotherapy;* 1975 Lea & Febiger
- Johnson, A.C., *Principles and Practice of Drugless Therapeutics;* 3rd Ed., 1946 Chiropractic Educational Extension Bureau
- Kovacs, R., *Electrotherapy and Light Therapy;* 6th Ed., 1949 Lea & Febiger
- Krusen, F., *Physical Medicine;* 1941 W. B. Saunders Co.
- Clayton, E.R., *Actinotherapy and Diathermy for the Student;* 1939. Ballers, Tindall & Cox

PHOTOTHERAPY

LASER THERAPY

L

DESCRIPTION

In speaking of lasers, we are talking about low level laser therapy (LLLT)[7], also called "cold lasers" or "soft lasers". Lasers are also used at higher power for surgical use, and this does not concern us in the discussion of naturopathic physiotherapy.

Unlike most of the modalities in this book, there is of course no historical use of lasers in the "golden age" of Naturopathy. Nevertheless, lasers have found their way into naturopaths' hands over the years, particularly the ones trained in acupuncture. With the plethora of devices commercially available today, it is necessary to not only include mention of them but to explain the very real differences between true lasers and light-emitting diodes (LEDs) that are often referred to as "lasers".

True lasers are generators of coherent light, which produces the phenomenon known as "speckling". If you shine a therapeutic laser, or even a laser pointer, at a wall, you will see tiny bits of light seemingly dancing on their own, on the surface. If you shine an LED light on a wall, you will see no speckling; moreover, the beam will fan out the farther you are from the wall. The laser remains the same size because all its photons line up in single file.

While LED light does have some therapeutic effect, it is minute compared to laser light, and LED devices are better reserved for conditions that are too sensitive for laser stimulation, such as scar tissue and keloids, for some wounds, and for stimulating acupuncture points (some authorities believe that the points become insensitive after too much treatment with true lasers).

Therapeutic lasers have power outputs up to 500 milliwatts. By contrast, LED devices (although they may have clusters of many LEDs) have only an output of 20 milliwatts or less per diode.

---

[7] Also now being called Photobiomodulation Therapy (PBMT).

Many clinical studies have been done showing the failure of incoherent light in the form of LEDs when compared to laser. They can be found in the referenced works at the end of this section.

There are, however, infrared lasers, where the wavelength of the light is within the infrared part of the spectrum, typically from 700-800 nanometers (nm).

EQUIPMENT NEEDED
Lasers are classified (Classes I, II, IIIa, IIIb and IV) depending on the potential for causing cellular damage.Most low level lasers are Class III devices.
Wavelengths between 660 nm and 905 nm have the ability to penetrate skin, and soft/hard tissues. This light has a good effect on pain, inflammation and tissue repair.

There are continuous wave lasers and newer pulsed laser devices.   Besides the wavelength of coherent light in the laser, the pulsing adds therapeutic benefits of other, lower frequencies as well by rapidly turning on and off the beam. A popular frequency by users is 250 Hz, which is said to be generally anti-inflammatory and good for most conditions.   On the other hand, some feel that 10 Hz is the best frequency for any condition involving brain function. Low frequencies, like 50 Hz is said to be stimulatory while higher frequencies like 1000 Hz and higher are inhibitory or sedative.

Blue and green lasers (400-600 nm) are mostly absorbed into the skin and do not penetrate any deeper. If it is not a skin condition (eczema, psoriasis, or wounds) being treated, you will need a higher wavelength laser. At around 800-1200 nm, the beam penetrates deeper and is better for deep pain and inflammation. A 930 nm laser will penetrate into a fatty layer but will be absorbed there.   The water bound in the interstitial fluid and the cells will absorb a laser at 970 nm.
•
• Apollo™ lasers, made by Pivotal Health System, are a long established line. They are continuous wave lasers.
• Avant Systems™ has over 80 presets for pulsing. Many of them are sweep through a range of pulsing frequencies. This reduces the need to try an pick one perfect pulsing frequency.
• Lumix Systems™ are unique in that they combine a pulsing 910nm laser with a continuous wave 810nm. This is the best of both worlds. They offer programmable pulsing frequencies up to 100,000Hz. These dual wavelength systems are Class IV lasers.
• 3B Scientific™ sells acupuncture lasers from European sources.

EFFECTS AND PURPOSE

- Low level laser therapy (LLLT) is believed to affect the function of connective tissue cells (fibroblasts), accelerates connective tissue repair, and is anti-inflammatory in action.
- Laser therapy relieves pain by increasing beta endorphin levels, increases ACTH levels, increases phagocyte activity, and raises immunoglobulin levels.
- Laser therapy hastens granulation in healing wounds, particularly at 633 nm.
- Wavelength chosen can vary the effects; for example, lasers at 633 nm and 670 nm cause vasodilation, but lasers at 660 nm causes vasoconstriction. Peripheral nerve injury responds best to infrared lasers at 830 nm, less favorably to lasers at 660 nm, but not at all to 880 nm or 950 nm. This likely represents a type of tissue resonance effect.
- Pulsed lasers sometimes have even more specificity. The most commonly recommended preset pulsing frequencies include 2.5Hz, 10,Hz, , 50Hz, 100Hz and 250Hz, based on the manufacturers and on several studies.

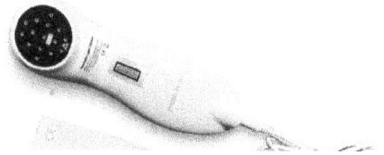
Cold laser with an array of lights

INDICATIONS FOR USE

- Pain
- Neuropathy
- Inflammation
- Slow healing wounds
- Connective tissue injuries

CONTRAINDICATIONS

- Implanted electronic devices such as pacemakers
- Pregnancy
- Do not treat over the thyroid gland.
- Do not treat over a gravid uterus.
- Do not treat over growth plates in young children
- Do not treat over neoplasms
- Never allow the beam to wander into the eyes

PRECAUTIONS

- Both operator and patient should wear protective eyewear.
- Glass objects, windows, and jewelry may reflect the laser beam. Environment for treatment should be examined with regard to this danger.
- Caution in treating epileptic patients with low-frequency pulsed lasers (visible pulsing might possibly induce seizure).

- Topical iodine (Betadine ™, etc.) on the skin can amplify laser penetration.
- Eating refined sugars and starches, in the form of seed oils, soft drinks, pastries, and white bread cause nitric oxide inhibition in the body, and lessen the effects of laser therapy.
-

ADVANTAGES
- Fairly rapid pain relief
- Inflammation reduction within hours or days
- Hastens tissue healing
- Good patient acceptance
- Painless
- Modern "high tech" reputation
- Low power (< 500 mw), Class III lasers have less potential for risk

DISADVANTAGES
- Cost of equipment
- Multiple devices may be needed if a wider variety of conditions are to be treated
- Lower power, Class III lasers as typically used by naturopaths have longer treatment times

INSTRUCTIONS
Treatment times vary from 20 seconds to 1 minute (depending on power of device).

1. Give patient protective goggles or otherwise protect vision.
2. Position patient for comfort.
3. Wash and dry areas to be treated.
4. Choose areas to treat based on four approaches:
   A. The site of injury (to promote healing, remodeling and reduce inflammation).
   B. Lymph nodes to reduce edema and inflammation.
   C. Nerves to induce analgesia.
   D. Trigger points to reduce tenderness and relax contracted muscle fibers.
   E. Acupuncture points according to meridian rationale
5. Apply laser to points according to case. One point or as many as 10-15 sites can be treated in a session.

   Dosage guide is on the following page.

TREATMENT DOSE GUIDE

(Based on Caucasian skin types—others may vary)

Conditions	Dose (Joule/Area)	Method	Time interval	Sessions
Acne Vulgaris	2 – 5 J / cm²	Spot treatment	2 – 3 days	4 – 10
Allergic rhinitis	4 -5 J / cm²	Spot treatment	2 – 3 days	5 – 10
Herpes simplex	4 -5 J / cm²	Spot treatment	Every day	2 – 3
Arthritis	4 -5 J / cm²	Spot treatment	2 – 3 days	8 – 10
Epicondylitis	4 -5 J / cm²	Spot treatment	2 – 3 days	8 – 10
Mucositis	4 -5 J / cm²	Spot treatment	2 – 3 days	5 – 10
Fibrositis	4 -5 J / cm²	Spot treatment	2 – 3 days	10 – 20
Hypersensitive teeth	4 -5 J / cm²	Spot treatment	2 – 3 days	5 – 10
Wound (edge)	4 -5 J / cm²	Spot treatment	2 – 3 days	3 – 10
Wound (open)	2 J / cm²	Hold 2 cm above	2 – 3 days	3 – 10
Scars and pregnancy	4 -5 J / cm²	Spot treatment	2 – 3 days	10 – 20
Nerve inflammation	4 -5 J / cm²	Spot treatment	2 – 3 days	5 – 10
Muscle knots and pain	5 – 50 J / point	Spot treatment	Every day (new injuries), max 3 days	
Muscle knots and pain	4 -5 J / cm²	Spot treatment	2 – 3 days	5 – 10
Pain (acute)	5 – 50 J / cm²	Spot treatment	Every day (new injuries), max 3 days	
Pain (subacute)	4 -5 J / cm²	Spot treatment	2 – 3 days	5 – 10
Arthritis, joints	4 -5 J / cm²	Spot treatment	2 – 3 days	10 – 15
Acupuncture, Reflexology	5 – 15 J / cm²	Spot treatment	2 – 3 days	3 – 10
Tendonitis	4 -5 J / cm²	Spot treatment	2 – 3 days	3 – 10
Removal of foot warts	5 – 10 J / point	Spot treatment	6 – 10 days	3 – 5
Trigger Points	5 -15 J / cm²	Spot treatment	2 – 3 days	
Tinnitus	50 – 300 J / ear	Spot treatment	2 – 3 days	10 – 20
Inflammation of the ear	50 – 300 J / ear	Spot treatment	2 – 3 days	2 – 3
Sinusitis	5 – 10 J / ear	Spot treatment	2 – 3 days	2 – 3
Sjögren Syndrome	5 – 10 J / ear	Spot treatment	2 – 3 days	3 – 10
Post Herpetic Neuralgia	5 – 10 J / ear	Spot treatment	2 – 3 days	3 – 10

FREQUENCY OF TREATMENT

Daily treatment for 2 weeks, or treatment every other day for 3-4 weeks, is recommended in most acute cases. Irradiation should cover most of the pathological tissue in the tendon or synovial tissue.

Start with energy dose in table, then reduce by 30% when inflammation is under control. The range of a therapeutic dose may range from +/- 50% of table values. Doses exceeding this are not considered <u>Low Level</u> Laser Therapy.

REFERENCES

- Michlovitz, S., *Thermal Agents in Rehabilitation,* 3rd Ed.; 1996 F.A. Davis Co.
- Akeda Laser ApS, Denmark

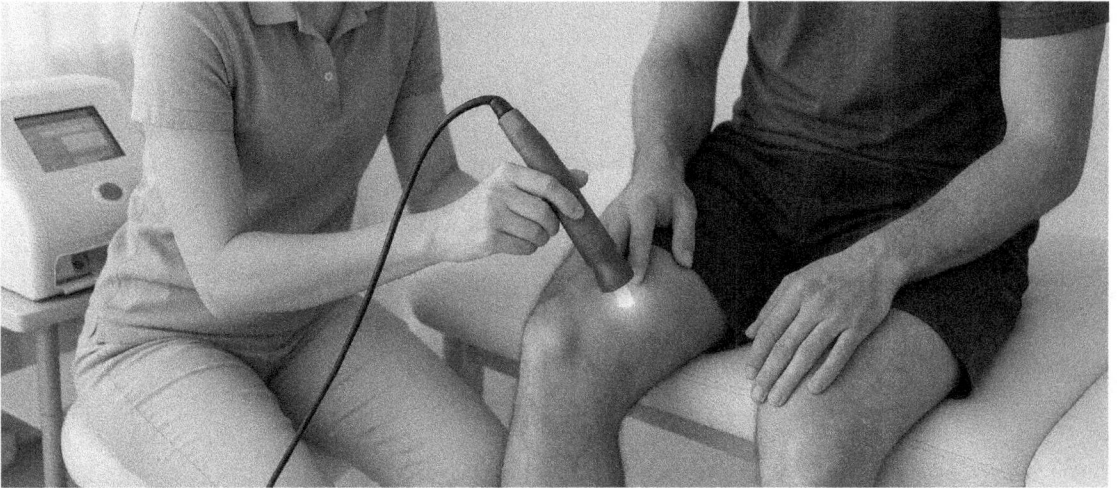

6

ELECTROTHERAPY

OVERVIEW

E

DESCRIPTION

Electrotherapy: The use of electricity for therapeutic purposes.
This sounds like a fairly simple matter to explain. It is not. The various types of electrical stimulation that have been traditionally used are confusing at first sight. Certain types are more suited for a given use than others. One may be effective for increasing tone in a weak muscle while another is better for relieving pain. The reader should consult the indications in each section to choose the most appropriate therapy for the case at hand.

Terminology has changed a bit over the past decades and we have included it wherever it differs from the traditional. Unipolar galvanic is now called "monophasic" and bipolar is called "biphasic". Much of electrical stimulation is now being referred to as "TENS" (transcutaneous electrical nerve stimulation) in spite of the fact that true TENS units produce frequencies and use wave forms that are unlike traditional electrotherapy. We are not covering conventional mode TENS, burst mode TENS, modulation mode TENS , nor Interferential Stimulation in this work.

More recent developments have increased both the complexity of the practice and the cost of the equipment. Some feel modern developments have also reduced the effectiveness in some areas. Whether an intended or an accidental byproduct, the advances and miniaturization in electronic technology has changed the field. Nevertheless, *the natural, physical characteristics of the various types of electricity remain the same, and their effects remain the same*. Naturopathic doctors can apply them in the same manner as their counterparts a hundred years ago and still achieve the same effects.

TYPES OF ELECTRICAL CURRENT

It is common to first separate two categories of equipment: "Low Volt" and "High Volt".

Low Volt

Low Volt devices deliver a number of different currents with a low voltage generator (below 100 volts) producing them. They are also called "low frequency" devices because they typically only generate frequencies of 1-10 Hz (pulses per second). Low frequency stimulation has been called "Acupuncture-like TENS", because it creates physiological responses similar to needle acupuncture. Chiropractors using low frequency electrotherapy currently call it EMS, for Electrical Muscle Stimulation, or simply "e-stim", or "muscle stim". Note: Real TENS devices are low voltage but generate higher frequencies (over 50 Hz, up to 110 Hz).

Low volt devices typically produce three types of current, traditionally called Faradic, Galvanic, and sinusoidal. These will be covered individually.

High Volt

High voltage machines became more prominent in the last few decades. Often called HVPC (High Voltage Pulsed Current), they usually have a maximum voltage of 150 volts but some as high as 500 volts. Most have a maximum peak current exceeding 80 milliamps, but for the higher voltage machines, as high as 2 amperes. They typically have a frequency range of 1 Hz to 125 Hz.

High volt devices have become popular in Physical Therapy due to the fact that the current is smoother and causes less patient sensation and thus less discomfort. Studies have shown that it is a bit better in treating sprains, tendonitis, and myofascitis than low volt machines. However, they seem to be inferior to low volt machines in treating muscle spasms, muscle re-education, and toning.

In general, low volt machines are most applicable to naturopathic practice and most supported by the naturopathic literature. **Therefore, all instructions hereafter apply to low volt devices.**

TYPES OF CURRENT AND WAVEFORMS

The physical characteristics of a therapeutic current are direction of flow and the shape or waveform.

MONOPHASIC

Monophasic or unidirectional currents flow in one direction only, with no reversal of polarity; that is, the polarity of one lead from the device is positive and the other is negative polarity. In the non-therapeutic realm this is referred to as direct current (DC). Monophasic current will not contract normal skeletal muscles. *Monophasic current has a chemical action while the other forms do not*, which will be discussed in depth in the **Monophasic** and **Ionization** sections[1].

Note how the impulses remain on the positive (+) side of the median line.

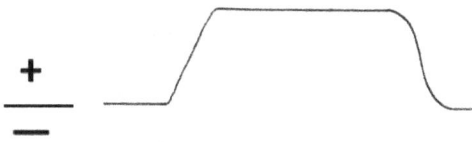

STRAIGHT GALVANIC   PULSED GALVANIC

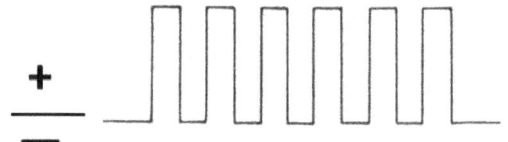

BIPHASIC

Biphasic or bidirectional currents reverse their direction of flow at a rate according to the frequency setting.   In the non-therapeutic realm this is referred to as alternating current (AC). It has no polarity effects as does the monophasic.

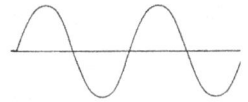

FARADIC

Faradic current causes strong contractions while biphasic current contracts more mildly. Faradic or biphasic are traditionally chosen for the strength of contraction desired for a condition.

Note on the next page how the faradic waveform has just a slight dip into the negative polarity while the biphasic waveform swings fully into each alternating polarity. Because of the relative similarity to a sine curve, this has been historically referred to as a sine wave current (although a sine waveform can be generated by a monophasic apparatus, such is actually referred to as "sinusoidal". The "sine wave" traditionally

---

[1] Static electricity is a unipolar current no longer used therapeutically and will not be included here.

used for therapy is a biphasic waveform). "Surging" denotes a current strength that rises, falls, and then has a period of rest, causing periodic muscle contractions.

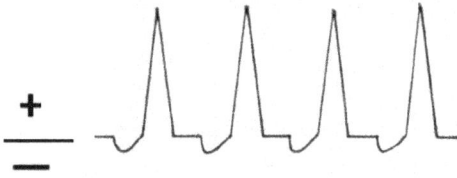

FARADIC

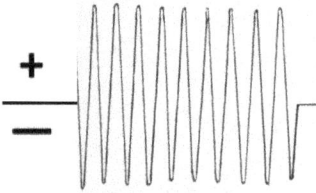

BIPHASIC

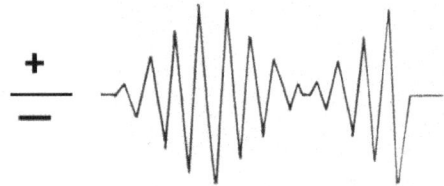

SURGING BIPHASIC

Other waveforms have come to be used in physiotherapy in modern times, such as the square wave, sawtooth wave, and triangle wave, all based on their appearance on an oscillograph. While they are used in contemporary therapy, they are not included here as they are somewhat superfluous for the beginning naturopath and have not made themselves indispensable for routine therapy.

FREQUENCY
In addition to type of current and waveform, the frequency by which they are repeated have therapeutic effects of their own. Low frequencies are measured in pulses per second (PPS) or Hertz (Hz). 1 Hz equals one pulse per second. Beginning with the work of Rife in the 1930s, specific frequencies have been found to resonate with specific conditions and even specific tissues. Consult a text on "frequency specific therapy" for more information that can introduce another aspect to your treatment.

ELECTRODIAGNOSIS
For completeness, electrodiagnosis should be mentioned. This is using electrical stimulation to evaluate the anatomical and electrical changes in the muscles or nerves that may have occurred due to an injury. As a result of that injury, the muscle may have become detached from its corresponding nerve. This is referred to as RD, or Reaction of

Degeneration, and has been traditionally evaluated by stimulation of the muscle with electricity (faradic or galvanic) to see how much stimulation it takes for a reaction. This practice has been mostly abandoned with the advent of newer, more sophisticated methods and developments in neurology. Assessment of such injuries should be referred to a neurologist.

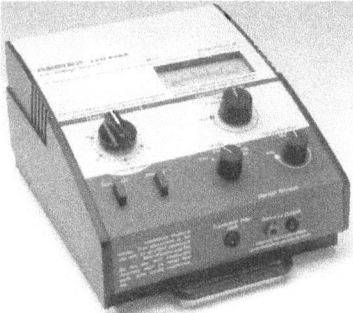

Amrex galvanic
monophasic unit

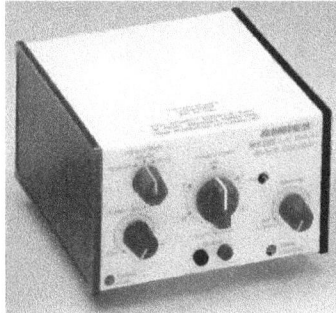

Amrex sine wave
biphasic unit

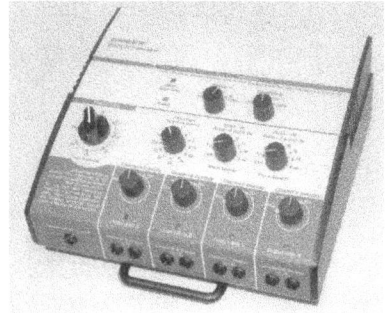

Amrex dual monophasic-
biphasic unit

Amrex® stimulators courtesy of amrexusa.com

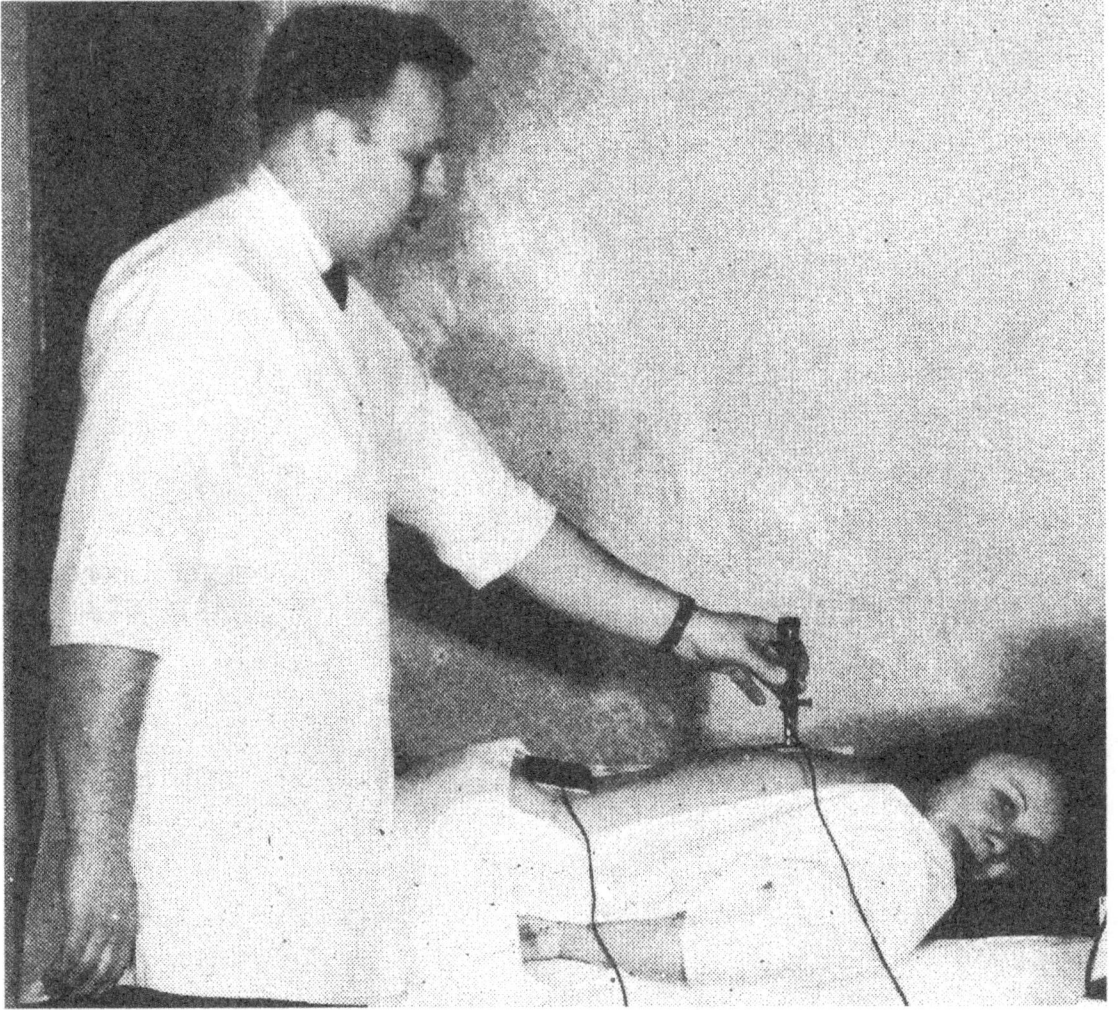

Alton C. Johnson, ND applies electrospinal therapy to a patient, ca. 1946.

ELECTROTHERAPY

FARADIC

E

DESCRIPTION

Faradic current is a spiked biphasic waveform that is asymmetrical. It has high peaks of short duration (0.1 to 1 millisecond). For this reason, it is very effective for producing nerve and muscle response. The frequency range is typically 50-100 Hz. It is usually applied in a surging wave, which creates a more natural rhythm of muscle contraction and relaxation. The surge period and rest period can be adjusted, usually surging from 2-5 seconds and then a rest cycle of 10-15 seconds.

EQUIPMENT NEEDED

This therapeutic current has been largely abandoned by conventional physiotherapy in the USA to the extent that electrotherapy equipment with multiple settings often do not include faradic stimulation. However, in recent years a popular use has arisen in the cosmetic field, under the name of Neuromuscular Electrical Stimulation (NMES). This is the use of faradic current for reduction of facial wrinkles and body toning. An apparatus that can produce faradic current is useful and worth having for other reasons. New Life Care in India makes a faradic instrument. A small unit with both faradic and galvanic (monophasic) settings is made by Acco™.

EFFECTS AND PURPOSE

- Mild analgesia by stimulating sensory nerves
- Triggers involuntary muscle contractions, useful for rehabilitation, muscle strengthening,
- Prevents muscles wasting while immobilized or unable to move without pain
- Restores impaired voluntary movement due to stroke or spinal cord injury
- Passive exercise for lax structures
- Promotes lymphatic drainage, aiding detoxification
- Increases blood flow
- Breaks down adhesions

INDICATIONS FOR USE
- Bell's Palsy
- Fibromyalgia and myofascial trigger points
- Back and neck pain due to muscle spasm
- Acute sciatica
- Discogenic pain with radiculopathy
- Loss of tone and muscle degeneration
- Spasticity
- Flat feet (pes planus)
- Rectal prolapse
- Pelvic floor stimulation
- Breast cancer-related lymphedema

CONTRAINDICATIONS
- Do not apply over the chest or heart region in patients with pacemakers
- Do not apply in arrhythmias, or other cardiac conditions
- Do not apply during pregnancy
- Do not apply over abdominal and pelvic areas
- Do not apply over open wounds, skin infections
- Do not apply over areas with severe neurological damage.
- Do not apply over areas with cancerous tumors.

PRECAUTIONS
- Proper electrode placement with regard to **motor points** is essential.
- Intensity of current must be monitored and within tolerance.
- Caution in applying to the neck or near the head in epileptic patients.

ADVANTAGES
- Simple procedure
- Short duration treatment session

DISADVANTAGES
- Requires steady treatments over several weeks for noticeable results
- Patients can feel a prickling that might not be pleasant

INSTRUCTIONS
1. Explain the procedure to the patient first.
2. Place one electrode pad over the site of the lesion or pain.

3. Place the other electrode pad distally on the affected extremity over the motor points of the affected muscle/nerve (see motor points chart elsewhere).
4. Use surging mode faradic stimulation at 10 milliamps (mA) intensity. The correct intensity should cause a visible muscle contraction (tetany). Surge rate should be 2-5 seconds, followed by 10-15 seconds rest.
5. Treat for 10 minutes, monitoring patient's tolerance.
6. If treating Bell's Palsy, place one electrode pad over the scapula and use a pencil electrode or cotton swab electrode to stimulate the motor points on the slack side of the face. Use about 2 mA of current for 2 minutes per point.

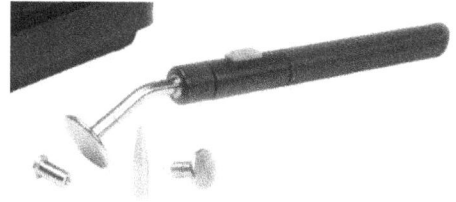

Mettler pencil electrode

FREQUENCY OF TREATMENT
2-5 treatments weekly; daily if possible at outset of therapy

REFERENCES

- Kovacs, R., *Electrotherapy and Light Therapy*; 6th Ed., 1949 Lea & Febiger
- Johnson, A.C., *Principles and Practice of Drugless Therapeutics*; 3rd Ed., 1946 Chiropractic Educational Extension Bureau
- Handbook of Physical Medicine; 1945 American Medical Association
- Morse, F., *Low Volt Currents of Physiotherapy*; 1925 General X-Ray Co.

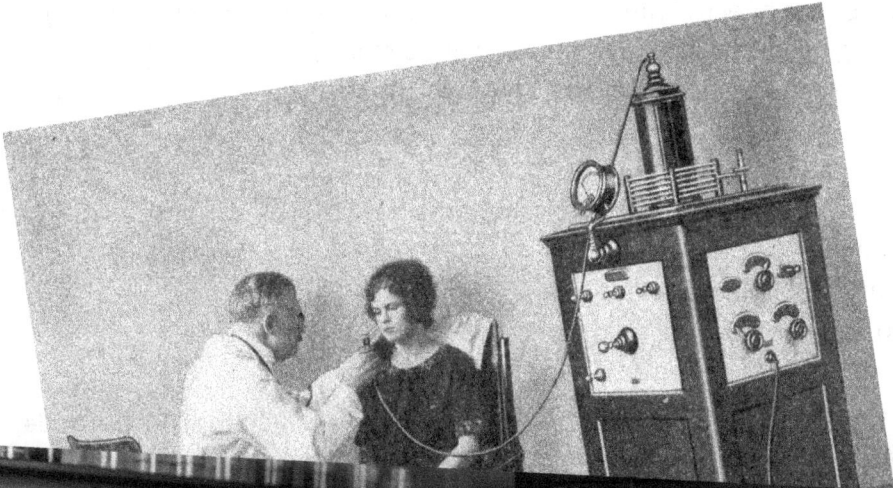

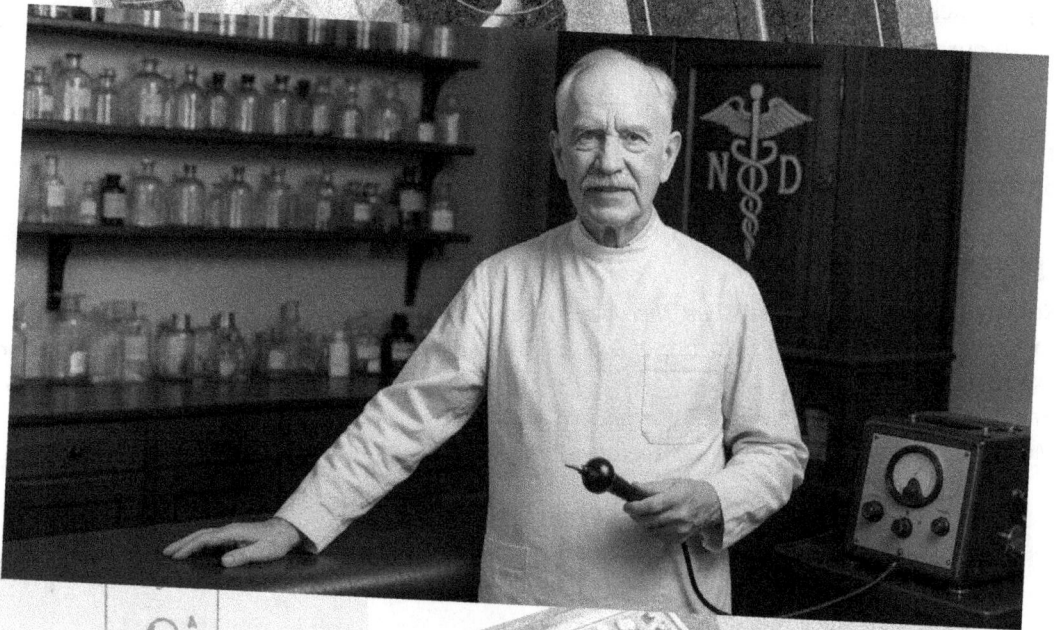

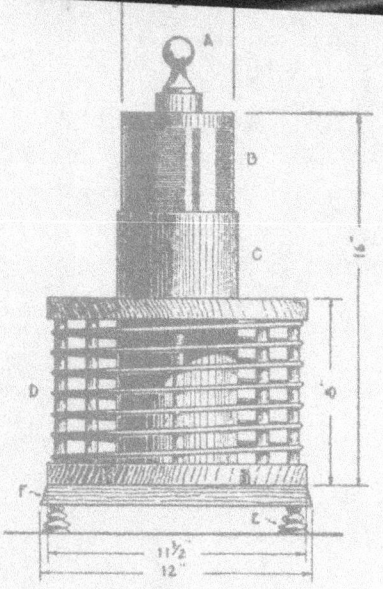

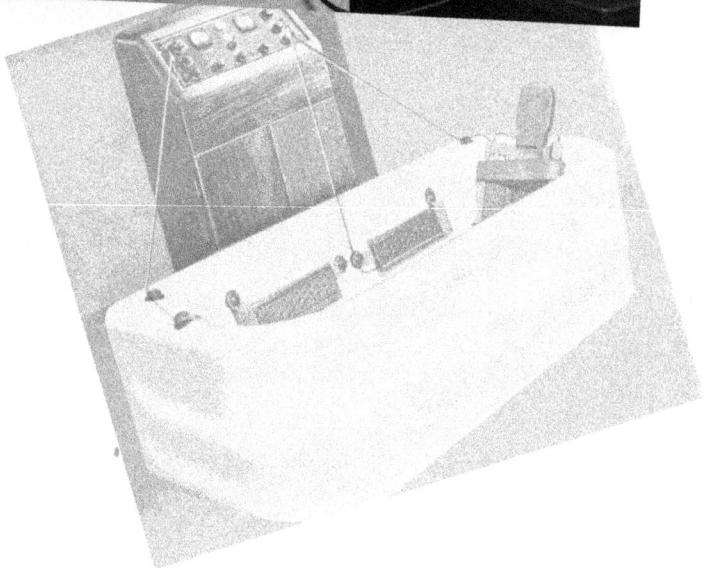

ELECTROTHERAPY

MONOPHASIC / UNIPOLAR (Galvanic)

E

DESCRIPTION

This is a ripple-free direct current so smooth that it will appear as a straight line on an oscillograph. Galvanic or unipolar current is also sometimes referred to as a "chemical current", as will be discussed in detail in the section on **Ion Transfer**. Unipolar current has the ability to cause chemical changes, unlike other types of current.

The basic rules are:
- The two electrodes in contact with the patient's body will have opposite polarities.
- The one you are using at the treatment site will be considered the active electrode.
- The other electrode that completes the circuit is called the indifferent or dispersive electrode.
- Use the positive pole at the site if you want to sedate a muscle or nerve
- Use the negative pole if you want to stimulate a muscle or nerve
- The smaller the electrode at the site of treatment, the greater the effect (sedation or stimulation)

EQUIPMENT NEEDED

There is a confusing array of devices available today. It is important to be clear that the apparatus you choose in fact produces a unipolar or monophasic current. TENS units do not.
One company still producing such equipment (and still refers to it as "galvanic") is Amrex.

EFFECTS AND PURPOSE

This type of electrotherapy is a direct current that travels from the positive pole to the negative pole; one direction only. It has three possible applications:

1. Anti-inflammatory action and pain relief;
2. Ionization: the introduction of medicinal substances into the tissues;
3. Electrolysis: chemical destruction of tissue (warts, fibroma, etc.) by concentration of the galvanic current at one small point.

The monophasic or galvanic current is probably more effective in relieving pain than biphasic current.

INDICATIONS FOR USE
- Pain of either acute or chronic nature
- Pain due to neuritis and neuralgia, peripheral nerve injuries
- Pain and swelling of injuries
- Inflammatory conditions
- Muscular fatigue
- Bursitis
- Edema
- Fibrosis
- Scars
- Chilblains
- Indolent wounds (for which use negative as the active electrode)

CONTRAINDICATIONS
- In the region of pacemakers or other implanted electronics
- Over superficial metal implants
- Over scars or wounds
- Over areas where active motion would be inadvisable (recently sutured tissues, fractures, etc.)
- Patients with myocardial weakness

PRECAUTIONS
Never place the electrodes or pads in a position that the current path runs through the cardiac region.

ADVANTAGES
- Non-invasive
- Effective pain relief
- Minimal training needed to perform
- Price of equipment can be moderate

DISADVANTAGES
Must navigate cables connecting patient to machine

INSTRUCTIONS
1. Explain the procedure to the patient. Describe the sensations likely to be felt.
2. Check the skin condition at the chosen treatment site. If the skin at the site is oily or has cosmetics on it, wash with soap and water before commencing treatment.
3. If the skin is cold, warm it first to increase circulation and perspiration, which help conductivity of the electricity. Hot pack or infrared are typically used, for 5 minutes.
4. Position patient so that you have complete access to the area under treatment.
5. Verify that the machine is not turned on before you place the electrodes.
6. Place the electrodes or pads according to desired effect: Positive (+) at a site of pain, congestion, or inflammation; negative (-) at a site of lax tissues, muscle atrophy, or reduced blood supply.
7. To ensure that they do not move, fix the pads with straps, weights, or use adhesive electrodes.
8. The electrode at the treatment site is considered the active electrode; the other is a dispersive or "indifferent" electrode. The treatment effect is more powerful if the active electrode is smaller than the indifferent.
9. With pads in place, connect cables to the machine.
10. Turn on the machine, set desired frequency, and slowly turn up the intensity, asking the patient to report when the tingling becomes uncomfortably strong. Immediately turn down the intensity to a tolerable setting. Rule of thumb is <u>1-2 milliamperes per square inch of active electrode size</u>.
11. Never change frequency settings or position of pads while the machine is running.
12. Apply the current (straight galvanic, pulsed galvanic, or surging) for 10 minutes.
13. Return controls to zero, switch machine off, and only then remove the pads.

FREQUENCY OF TREATMENT
According to need. Once or twice a week in conjunction with other therapies if possible.

REFERENCES
- Kovacs, R., *Electrotherapy and Light Therapy*; 6th Ed., 1949 Lea & Febiger
- Krusen, F., *Physical Medicine*; 1941 W. B. Saunders Co.
- Johnson, A.C., *Principles and Practice of Drugless Therapeutics*; 3rd Ed., 1946 Chiropractic Educational Extension Bureau
- *Handbook of Physical Medicine*; 1945 American Medical Association

GALVANIC CURRENT

POSITIVE (+)	NEGATIVE. (-)
Produces oxygen	Produces hydrogen
Attracts acids	Attracts alkali
Repels alkali	Repels acid
Hardens tissue	Softens tissue
Contracts tissue	Dilates tissue
Vasoconstrictor	Vasodilator
Stops hemorrhage	Increases hemorrhage
Reduces congestion	Increases congestion
Sedative	Stimulating
Relieves pain in acute conditions (reduction of congestion)	Reduces pain in chronic conditions (softens tissues and increases circulation)

ELECTROTHERAPY

IONIZATION

DESCRIPTION

Iontophoresis[2] is the technical term for the transfer of medicinal solutions from the surface of the skin to the inner tissues. Gould's Medical Dictionary defines it as "The introduction of ions into the body by electric current, for therapeutic purposes". In mainstream medicine, this is often referred to as "ionic medication". <u>This is of profound significance for a naturopath who is philosophically or legally not able to perform injections.</u>

Ionization is done with the use of galvanic (monophasic) current, as discussed in the previous section. It is made possible due to a phenomenon of physics, where an atom or molecule that has a positive or negative charge (an *ion*) is repelled by a force of the same polarity.

Galvanic electricity, as it passes through the body, breaks up some molecules into their component atoms, releasing polarized ions, which have either a positive or negative charge. This is the reason for the different effects of the current, as alluded to in the **Monophasic** section. By applying the correct polarity in therapy (by the active electrode), one achieves these effects:

Positive ions are driven by the positive pole. Negative ions are driven by the negative pole.

A solution that is positively charged will be driven into the tissues by the positive polarity current.

A solution that is negatively charged will be driven into the tissues by the negative polarity current.

---

[2] Also called *cataphoresis*.

As examples of the polarity of different substances, these possess a positive charge (and are thus driven by the positive pole): magnesium, sulfur, iron, silver, zinc, copper, quinine, and also adrenaline and cocaine.

Those possessing a negative charge (and are thus driven by the negative pole) include: acetic acid, potassium, iodine ions, chlorine ions, salicylate ions.

"Ions" in the sentence above is emphasized because of their ability to render an element polarized in combination. For example, elemental sodium itself is neutral, but combined with chloride ions to make sodium chloride, it becomes negative.

Important for naturopaths: While many are neutral, some plant extracts have a polarity, such as white willow (-). With its proven ability to fight pain and inflammation, ionization of this plant extract is a useful tool. Or Calendula (+), with its healing power on the skin. Vitamins have even been successfully ionized in certain conditions[3]. Some of the solutions typically used in ionization are listed here in their strengths.

To make a given solution:

2 oz. of the mineral salt or plant tincture/fluid extract, plus 20 oz. water = 10% solution.
One part 10% solution to 9 parts water = 1% solution.
Two parts 10% solution to 8 parts water = 2% solution.

Add one ounce of the 2% solution to 7 ounces of warm water at the time of application.

---

[3] Rong S., Wang C., Han B., Feng P., Lan W., Gao Z., Li X., Chen W. Iontophoresis-assisted accelerated riboflavin/ultraviolet A scleral cross-linking: A potential treatment for pathologic myopia. Exp. Eye Res. 2017;162:37–47. doi: 10.1016/j.exer.2017.07.002.

Lombardo M., Giannini D., Lombardo G., Serrao S. Randomized controlled trial comparing transepithelial corneal cross-linking using iontophoresis with the Dresden Protocol in progressive keratoconus. Ophthalmology. 2017;124:804–812. doi: 10.1016/j.ophtha.2017.01.040.

ION SOLUTIONS

Iodine solution (-)	1 part Lugol's to 3 parts water
Potassium iodide (-)	1.5%
Potassium citrate (-)	2%
Sodium salicylate (-)	1% - 2%
Sodium chloride (-)	2%
Copper sulfate (+)	1% - 2%
Lithium carbonate. (+)	1%
Lithium chloride (+)	2%
Zinc sulfate. (+)	1% - 2%
Acetic acid (+)	5%
Magnesium sulfate (+)	2%
Salix alba (white willow) (-)	2%
Hypericum (St. John's wort) (-)	2%
Calendula officinalis (+)	2%

EQUIPMENT NEEDED

- A **monophasic** (unipolar) stimulator capable of delivering galvanic DC current, is essential. See previous section. Modern devices have a variety of programs; <u>be sure to choose a "constant" setting</u>.
- Ionic solutions according to the condition being treated.
- Large and small electrodes

Note: The electrode material is a considerable factor during ionization. For best results, the most recommended type is silver or silver chloride (Ag/AgCl) surfaced electrodes, which can resist changes in pH. Inert electrode materials, on the other hand (platinum, stainless steel), use water, can alter the solution's pH and can lead to degradation of proteins and peptides. Physical therapy suppliers carry iontophoretic patches, which are ideal for this method. Nevertheless, ionization has been successfully used for decades before the introduction of specific electrodes as described.

EFFECTS AND PURPOSE

Dual therapy combining the known benefit of galvanic stimulation with the enhanced absorption of medicinal substances for local or even systemic effect.

INDICATIONS FOR USE

- Pain and inflammation
- Rheumatoid arthritis
- Gout
- Rhinitis
- Plantar warts
- Athlete's foot and other topical fungal infections
- Decubitus ulcer

CONTRAINDICATIONS

- Should not be used in pregnancy;
- Should not be used during lactation;
- Hypersensitivity to the active substance
- Metal implanted close to the skin surface in the area treated
- Recent scars in the area treated
- Patients with cardiac pacemakers

PRECAUTIONS

Ensure that there is no anesthetic skin in the target area.

ADVANTAGES

- Non-invasive
- Places within the hands of the naturopath the advantages of injection
- Substances may be absorbed that are difficult to take by mouth
- Relatively short treatment times

DISADVANTAGES

- Need for preparation of solutions initially

INSTRUCTIONS

1. Explain the procedure to the patient. Describe the sensations likely to be felt.
2. Check the skin condition at the chosen treatment site. If the skin at the site is oily or has cosmetics on it, wash with soap and water before commencing treatment.
3. If the skin is cold, warm it first to increase circulation and perspiration, which help conductivity of the electricity. Hot pack or infrared are typically used, for 5 minutes.
4. Position patient so that you have complete access to the area under treatment.
5. Verify that the machine is not turned on before you place the electrodes.
6. Select smaller electrode for the active and a larger for the indifferent.
7. Moisten active electrode with the chosen solution and place at the target site. It should be thoroughly moist but not dripping.
8. Place larger indifferent electrode at a convenient site on the skin on the same side of the body, but a greater distance away than the width of the electrode itself.
9. To ensure that they do not move, fix the pads with straps, weights, or use adhesive electrodes.
10. With pads in place, connect cables to the machine. <u>Be certain to connect the active electrode to the appropriate polarity for the solution on the pad</u>. Note: The convention is for the positive cable to be <u>red</u> and the negative cable <u>black</u>.
11. Turn on the machine, set for continuous galvanic, and set intensity to within patient tolerance (usual formula is 1-2 milliamperes per square inch of active electrode size). Usual dose is 40 milliampere minutes (4 mA for 10 minutes, or 2 mA for 20 minutes). Frequency is not relevant.
12. Never change wave settings or position of pads while the machine is running.
13. Apply the current (straight galvanic) for 15-20 minutes.
14. Return controls to zero, switch machine off, and only then remove the pads.
15. Clean the surface of the skin where the electrodes were and dry the patient.

FREQUENCY OF TREATMENT

Refer to specific treatment protocols following.

IONIZATION PROTOCOLS

All treatments use straight, <u>non-surging</u> galvanic current.

Athlete's foot, trichophyton infection	Fill basin with 2% copper sulfate solution (+). Immerse foot and drop in the tip of the positive cable to the solution. Place larger pad on calf, connect to negative pole. Use 2- 2.5 milliamps current per square inch of pad, or to tolerance, 15 minutes twice weekly. Sometimes only a few sessions will clear the condition.
Boils	Soak active electrode (-)in white willow bark solution or sodium salicylate solution, 2%. Ideally, paint the target area with tincture of iodine prior. Treat at 5-10 milliamperes for 6 minutes, twice weekly.
Bursitis	Active electrode (+) soaked in 2% Magnesium sulfate solution. Secure over the anterior shoulder, larger indifferent electrode on posterior shoulder. Treat to tolerance for 10-20 minutes, twice weekly
Decubitus ulcer	Active electrode (+) soaked in 2% zinc sulfate solution (or mixed in gel), or combined with Calendula solution 2%, treat to tolerance for 20 minutes, weekly for 2-3 weeks
Fungal infections	Active electrode (+) soaked with 2% copper sulfate solution. Use 2- 2.5 milliamperes current per square inch of pad, or to tolerance, 15 minutes twice weekly. Sometimes only a few sessions will clear the condition.
Goiter, adolescent (non-cystic)	3 x 3 electrode soaked in warm potassium iodide 2% solution is the active electrode, negative (-). Larger indifferent electrode between scapulae, positive (+). Treat at 5-8 milliamperes x 15 minutes, twice weekly.
Gout	Soak active electrode (+) in lithium carbonate or lithium chloride 2% solution. Treat to tolerance for 20 minutes, weekly x 4 weeks.
Inflammation, acute and subacute	Soak active electrode (-)in white willow bark solution or sodium salicylate solution, 2%, or combine with Hypericum solution 2%. Treat to tolerance for 15-20 minutes.
Plantar warts	Soak active electrode (-) in white willow bark solution or sodium salicylate solution, 2%. Treat at 10 milliamperes for 10-15 minutes weekly.
Rheumatoid arthritis	Soak active electrode in sodium citrate solution 2%. Apply to target joint and treat at 7-10 milliamperes for 20 minutes, 3 times weekly in acute phase.
Rhinitis and sinusitis (frontal or maxillary)	Mix 2% zinc sulfate solution into a neutral gel, coat cotton tampon and insert into nostril. Connect to positive (+) cable using a clip. Indifferent electrode on the back of the neck. Treat at 3 milliamperes for 3 minutes. Repeat with the other nostril.

Sinusitis, sphenoid	Same technic as for rhinitis but use 2% copper sulfate solution instead.

These protocols can also be used with ultrasound in the place of galvanic stimulation. See **Phonophoresis** section elsewhere.

REFERENCES

- Hayes, K., *Manual for Physical Agents;* 4th Ed., 1984 Appleton & Lange
- Fischer, R.A., *Low Volt Currents used in Physical Therapy;* 1965 R.A. Fischer & Co.
- Kovacs, R., *Electrotherapy and Light Therapy*; 6th Ed., 1949 Lea & Febiger
- Johnson, A.C., *Principles and Practice of Drugless Therapeutics*; 3rd Ed., 1946 Chiropractic Educational Extension Bureau
- Krusen, F., *Physical Medicine*; 1941 W. B. Saunders Co.
- Handbook of Physical Medicine; 1945 American Medical Association

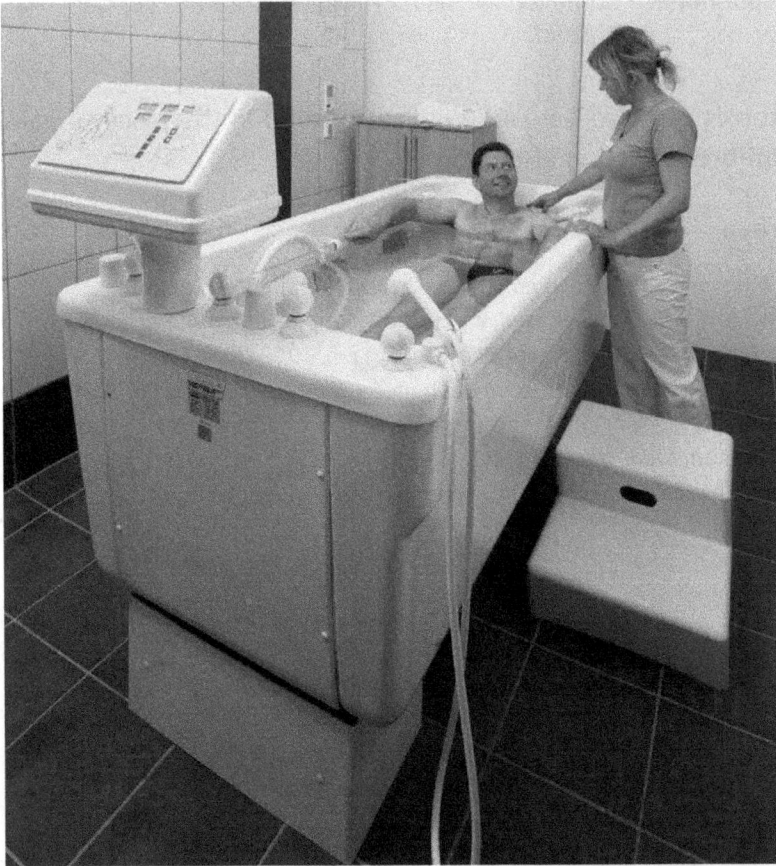

German naturopathic clinics offer the **Stanger Bath**, a form of ionization mixed with hydrotherapy. Herbal-mineral solutions are dissolved in the bath water and the galvanic current drives the medicinal compounds into the tissues.

ELECTROTHERAPY

BIPHASIC / BIPOLAR (sine wave)

E

DESCRIPTION

An alternating electrical current (AC) that alternates between positive polarity and negative polarity in quick succession. Because early devices produced an actual rounded sine curve, this used to be referred to as "sine wave" current. Today, the wave produced by modern components is usually a square shape but still sometimes referred to as a sine wave. Low volt devices in this category operate with a voltage range of 20-35 volts, and the pulse width (durations) is usually set to 50% of the maximum voltage of the particular device. Muscle stimulation by a biphasic current is basically done by placing electrodes on the skin, connecting them by cables to the stimulator, and applying a tolerable current that produces some degree of muscle contraction. By adjusting the output ,you can create different effects.

Currently, biphasic machines are commonly called "electrical muscle stimulators" (EMS), because that is their main use in standard Physical Therapy. EMS units transmit electrical impulses through the skin that stimulate the nerves in the treatment area. This creates involuntary muscle contractions, useful for relaxing spasm, relieving pain, and restoring range of motion. While naturopaths have used this current to affect organic processes as well, Physical Therapy does not do this, as a rule. An emphasis in recent years has been to use EMS on incapacitated patients to improve or maintain muscle tone without actual physical activity. This is likely because stroke and its residual atrophy and spasticity has become more common.

Many uses for biphasic current are best applied in what has traditionally been called "surging sine wave". The is, in modern parlance, a "ramped" bipolar current: an alternating wave that rhythmically increases and decreases in intensity. Some conditions call for a slow surge, some for a rapid surge, so the rate or frequency can be set accordingly on the machine. The surging or "ramped" current more closely

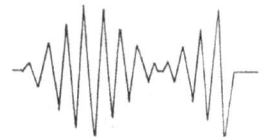

resembles a natural muscle contraction and therefore creates a smoother stimulation of the muscle fibers.

Obviously, there are no polarity effects from this current as there is in **monophasic** (galvanic) current, because anything the positive pulse would do, the negative pulse would immediately undo, and vice-versa. So biphasic current has no chemical effects and cannot be used for ionization.

EQUIPMENT NEEDED

One needs an EMS stimulator. Some devices are dual TENS/EMS combination units, but you must have a device that says it is "EMS". While professional models are marketed to physical therapists, one can buy a small and portable —and completely effective—device online for very little money. These are battery-operated units, and they can serve well in a clinical setting.

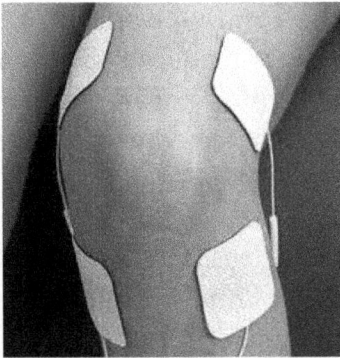

A two-channel device has the advantage of being able to stimulate four sites at once, as seen at left.

Some well-known companies producing electrotherapy equipment today include LGMedSupply, Amrex, Omron, HealthmateForever, iReliev, Pure Enrichment, and TechCare.

Two-channel treatment of knee

EFFECTS AND PURPOSE

The involuntary muscle contractions created by the biphasic (sine) current are useful for relaxing spasm, relieving pain, restoring range of motion, and restoring normal tone to viscera.

INDICATIONS FOR USE

- To increase local blood circulation
- Pain relief
- Relaxation of muscle spasms
- Reduction of atonic and also spastic constipation
- Maintaining or increasing range of motion
- Prevention or retardation of disuse atrophy
- Muscular re-education
- Immediate post-surgical stimulation of calf muscles to prevent venous thrombosis

CONTRAINDICATIONS

- In the region of pacemakers or other implanted electronics
- Over superficial metal implants
- Over scars or wounds
- Over areas where active motion would be inadvisable (recently sutured tissues, fractures, etc.)
- Patients with myocardial weakness

PRECAUTIONS

Never place the electrodes or pads in a position that the current path runs through the cardiac region.

ADVANTAGES

- Non-invasive
- Effective pain relief
- Minimal training needed to perform
- Price of equipment can be moderate

DISADVANTAGES

Must navigate cables connecting patient to machine

INSTRUCTIONS

1. If it is desired that a muscle contract, a frequency setting of 30-50 Hz should be used. If nerve tissue is the target or pain relief is the goal, a higher frequency in the range of 80-110 Hz is used.
2. Explain the procedure to the patient. Describe the sensations likely to be felt.
3. Check the skin condition at the chosen treatment site. If the skin at the site is oily or has cosmetics on it, wash with soap and water before commencing treatment.
4. If the skin is cold, warm it first to increase circulation and perspiration, which help conductivity of the electricity. Hot pack or infrared are typically used, for 5 minutes.
5. Position patient so that you have complete access to the area under treatment.
6. Verify that the machine is not turned on before you place the electrodes.
7. Place the electrodes or pads according to desired effect:
   (a) over motor points over the muscles to be stimulated;
   (b) arranged proximal and distal to the affected area, so that the treatment current runs longitudinally through it;

(c) on the abdomen over both the ascending and descending colon, in the case of constipation (use slow rate of contraction);

(d) over the bladder and against the perineum for bladder problems, etc.

8. To ensure that they do not move, fix the pads with straps, weights, or use adhesive electrodes.

9. The electrode pads have equal power unless one is smaller. The smaller one, if used, should be located at the problem site and the other pad some distance from it (a distance at least the diameter of the pad itself). The treatment effect is more powerful at the smaller electrode.

10. With pads in place, connect cables to the machine.

11. Turn on the machine, set desired frequency, and slowly turn up the intensity, asking the patient to report when the tingling becomes uncomfortably strong. Immediately turn down the intensity to a tolerable setting. Only adjust the intensity during the rest periods if using interrupted biphasic (surging sine).

12. Never change frequency settings or position of pads while the machine is running.

13. Apply the current for 10 minutes for inhibition or relaxation. To stimulate, 6-8 contractions. For muscle re-education, a total of 10 contractions may be all that is needed.

14. Return controls to zero, switch machine off, and only then remove the pads.

FREQUENCY OF TREATMENT

As needed per the intensity of the symptoms, and the length of time they have been present.

Muscle re-education needs to be repeated twice a week.

REFERENCES

- Hayes, K., *Manual for Physical Agents;* 4th Ed., 1984 Appleton & Lange
- Kovacs, R., *Electrotherapy and Light Therapy;* 6th Ed., 1949 Lea & Febiger
- Johnson, A.C., *Principles and Practice of Drugless Therapeutics;* 3rd Ed., 1946 Chiropractic Educational Extension Bureau
- *Handbook of Physical Medicine;* 1945 American Medical Association
- Morse, F., *Low Volt Currents of Physiotherapy;* 1925 General X-Ray Co.

ELECTROTHERAPY

HIGH FREQUENCY PLASMA TUBE

E

DESCRIPTION

High Frequency Electrotherapy here refers to a different modality than a physical therapist or chiropractor would call "high frequency" (because diathermy and ultrasound generate frequencies in the megahertz range, they are referred to as "high frequency" devices). To the naturopathic doctor, this term refers to a device using a high frequency Tesla coil (HFTC). It produces a high voltage, high frequency, but low amperage current in the kilohertz range. This is projected into a glass vacuum tube or gas-filled tube. Electrically activating the gas inside the tube creates a "plasma" discharge.

The device consists of a wand that contains an Oudin-modified Tesla coil, connected to a resonance transformer with an adjustable spark gap. A glass tube with a metal connector is inserted into the wand and the current excites noble gases inside the tube to produce an "effleuve" (very fine sparks) discharge, or coarse sparks, depending on the gap between the tube and the skin. The tube is moved across the skin so that the current saturates the tissues. Sometimes it is lifted away from the skin to allow the sparks to jump from the tube to the skin surface, which produces a slightly different stimulation.

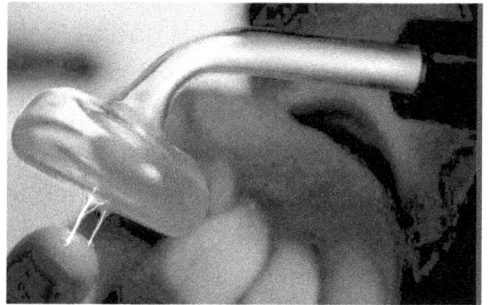
Effleuve.

EQUIPMENT NEEDED

This type of device is often sold as a "Violet Ray" wand. In the first half of the 20th Century, Violet Ray devices were widely touted for every kind of ailment and sold in the millions. This resulted in their being practically banned. The end result of this is that in the USA it is usually designated as a "quack" device. Other countries, particularly the Slavic countries, have continued to use and develop these instruments. This is not useless quackery. In the hands of a competent operator, it can do much good.

163

High frequency electrotherapy equipment can still be found today from companies such as Novator, Uupas, and FreqDance. Most modern units manufactured in the last 10-20 years have an output power of 15 Watts. The models of yesteryear had an output strength of 30 Watts—double the power. Consequently, the newer devices have been emphasized for cosmetic applications: acne, cellulite, wrinkle smoothing, etc. While the effect on the skin is very real, the newer models likely do not have the power to affect deeper tissues and viscera like the old ones. Hence, it is easy to "disprove" the claims made for the old Violet Ray of the past. There are some modern units with a 30 Watt output. Used older units can still be found and it may be to the naturopath's advantage to look for one as an addition to the natural physiotherapy armamentarium.

EFFECTS AND PURPOSE
- Create a mild hyperemia
- Increase temperature at the site
- Have a local germicidal action
- Increase local nutrition
- Increase tissue oxygenation
- Increase elimination of CO_2
- Increase elimination of metabolic waste products through the skin

Because the spark gap produces a wide range of randomly fluctuating frequencies, and also because the polarity of the current penetrating the body is alternating so rapidly, it has been speculated that the effect on the body is one of "cellular massage". This refers to the theory that each type of tissue's cells has an oscillatory rate that is unique to it. In illness, it deviates from that natural frequency. By being exposed to a variety of frequencies in close proximity, the sick tissue resonates with its signature frequency (picked out of the group, so to speak) and the cells begin oscillating normally again.

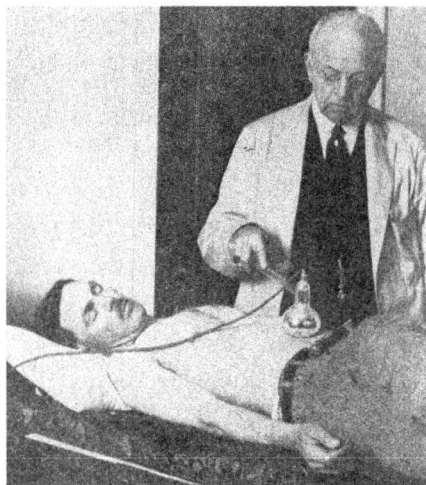

INDICATIONS FOR USE
- Surface infections
- Neuralgia and neuritis
- Lymphadenopathy
- Inflammation
- Acneform eruptions

CONTRAINDICATIONS
Open wounds

PRECAUTIONS
- Do not use around flammable substances; hair product, or alcohol-based gels, etc.
- Do not run the coil for more than ten minutes at a time without shutting off the machine to let it cool.

ADVANTAGES
Can be used over tender areas that cannot tolerate other types of stimulation

DISADVANTAGES
- Glass tubes must be handled with care
- Inadvertent (or deliberate) sparking of the skin is unsettling to many people

INSTRUCTIONS
1. Explain the procedure with an eye toward allaying fear of being "shocked".
2. Dust area to be treated with body powder.
3. Place the electrode against the skin before turning on the current, to avoid startling the patient.
4. Hold in firm contact with the skin during treatment, and move slowly over the area.
5. Applying the current to an area for 20-60 seconds is stimulative. Holding the glass electrode slightly off the skin and allowing the current to spark between skin and glass increases the stimulation. Sometimes creating a local erythema and a counter-irritating effect is used for conditions like alopecia, fibrositic, neuritis, ulcers, and acne.
6. Applying the current to an area for 2-5 minutes is inhibitive or sedative.

Moisture will create more drastic sparks against the skin, resulting possibly in an urticarial rash. For this reason, the powder serves both to insulate and lubricate.

FREQUENCY OF TREATMENT
Can be used daily if needed.

REFERENCES
- Johnson, A.C., *Principles and Practice of Drugless Therapeutics*; 3rd Ed., 1946 Chiropractic Educational Extension Bureau
- Krusen, F., Physical Medicine; 1941 W. B. Saunders Co.
- Eberhart, N.M., *Eberhart's Manual of High Frequency Currents*, 1926 New Medicine Pub. Co.
- Sampson, C. M., *Physiotherapy Technic;* 1923 Mosby Co.

ELECTROTHERAPY

SHORT WAVE DIATHERMY

E

DESCRIPTION

Diathermy (a term that literally means "heating through") is a type of electrotherapy using high frequency energy to heat deep tissues and produce a therapeutic response. Short Wave diathermy current is a high frequency alternating current. The heat energy obtained from the wave is used for giving relief to the patient. The standard frequency is 27.12 megahertz (27,120,000 cycles per second) and the wavelength is 11 meters.

There are two types of instruments: One uses two electrodes with the body part placed between them (dipole), historically referred to as "capacitive diathermy". The other has a coil that is aimed at the body part (monopole) and is usually referred to as "inductive diathermy". Both methods allow radio waves to pass into the tissues, rapidly oscillating the cells and heating them in the process. The pumping action draws new blood and nutrients into the tissues while speeding up the rate of expulsion of waste. This action is at the same time anti-inflammatory and a stimulant to healing, due to the increase in cell metabolism.

EQUIPMENT NEEDED

Machines available today come in 300-Watt and 500-Watt versions. The greater power of the 500-Watt version makes it a more reliable and effective choice. Modern diathermy units have both continuous and pulsed settings. Pulse frequencies can include 10 Hz, 20Hz, 50Hz, 100Hz, and 400 Hz. The pulse duration can range from 65 microseconds to 400 microseconds.

Many companies who used to manufacture short wave machines in the UAS no longer do so;

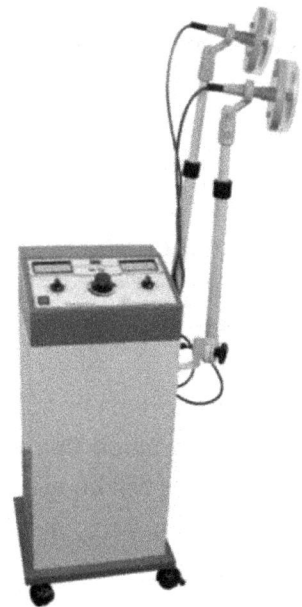

BTL's **MediLap** model diathermy

Mettler Electronics and **BTL Net** still do. **Siemens** in Germany, **MediChem Electronics** in India, and **Ito Physiotherapy** in Japan all make SWD devices.

EFFECTS AND PURPOSE

Short wave diathermy creates high frequency radio waves that vibrate the cells of the target tissues. This creates heat in the tissues, reducing congestion, inflammation, and pain in the muscles and other tissues, and accelerates the healing process of the damaged cells. Local metabolism is increased.

INDICATIONS FOR USE

- Subacute and chronic myofascial and musculoskeletal pain; Strains and sprains
- Sinusitis
- Joint stiffness
- Myospasm
- Tendonitis and tenosynovitis
- Bursitis
- Degenerative joint disease
- Arthritis
- Frozen shoulder
- Rehabilitation from injuries
- Congestion in the viscera
- Increases blood circulation
- Increases oxygenation and enhances nutritional uptake

CONTRAINDICATIONS

- Any metal in the treatment site that cannot be removed
- Pacemakers or any implanted metallic devices
- Acute inflammation
- Open wounds
- Over immature bone growth plates
- Over ischemic tissue
- Pregnancy
- Cancer
- Bleeding disorders or active bleeding
- Those taking blood thinning drugs
- Existing fever will be elevated

PRECAUTIONS

- Always question patient about metallic implants.

- Place toweling against the skin at the site of treatment to absorb sweat. Water heats up faster than skin and could burn the patient if allowed to collect.
- All electronics must be removed from the treatment area (cell phones, car keys, watches, computers, etc.,) or risk being damaged.

ADVANTAGES
- Non-invasive
- Cost effective compared to pharmaceutical treatment
- Effective pain relief
- Minimal training needed to perform

DISADVANTAGES
- Equipment is expensive
- Equipment takes up space

INSTRUCTIONS
General:

For pulsed diathermy units with variable frequency settings, these frequency ranges have been useful.

- Acute trauma, inflammation, or edema: 100-200Hz
- Subacute inflammation: 800Hz at 10 watts
- Pain reduction: 800Hz at 12 watts
- Spasm, chronic inflammation, to increase blood flow: 800Hz at 12 watts
- Stretching collagen-rich fibers: 800Hz at 48 watts

1. Explain the process to patient.
2. Have patient remove all metal and electronic devices (car keys, cell phone, credit cards with magnetic strip, etc.).
3. Inspect the skin at the treatment site for moisture. Dry it and apply Terry cloth towel to absorb any sweat that occurs.
4. Place patient on a non-metallic table or chair.
5. Position patient in a comfortable position allowing the machine to accurately aim at the treatment site. Explain that the patient should not move around once the treatment begins.
6. Try to position the machine so that the patient cannot disturb it.

Capacitance diathermy:
1. If using capacitance diathermy with two electrodes, they should be 1-3 inches from the body and even distances. If spacing is not equal, more heat will be produced under the electrode closest to the skin.
2. Electrodes should be parallel to skin surface, or it will create a "hot spot" where they are closer to the skin.
3. Electrodes should be farther from each other than the total spacing from the skin to the electrodes.
4. Patient should feel a mild warmth. Adjust power to avoid too much heat.
5. Treat for 20-30 minutes. Subacute inflammation should be treated for 10-15 minutes.

Induction diathermy:

1. If using induction diathermy with one drum electrode, it should be placed against toweling on the body at the treatment site.
2. If the unit tunes itself automatically, adjust the power so that the patient feels only a mild warmth.
3. If the unit requires manual tuning, turn the output control to 1/3 of the total power. Then adjust the tuning dial to tune the circuit to resonance with the patient. The needle on the gauge will rise and fall as you turn the dial. When it reaches its highest reading, the oscillator circuit is tuned. Keep that setting.
4. Treat for 20-30 minutes. Subacute inflammation should be treated for 10-15 minutes.

FREQUENCY OF TREATMENT

Daily if needed for subacute, less often for chronic.

REFERENCES

- Michlovitz, S., *Thermal Agents in Rehabilitation*, 3rd Ed.; 1996 F.A. Davis Co.
- Hayes, K., *Manual for Physical Agents;* 4th Ed., 1984 Appleton & Lange
- Kovacs, R., *Electrotherapy and Light Therapy*; 6th Ed., 1949 Lea & Febiger
- Johnson, A.C., *Principles and Practice of Drugless Therapeutics*; 3rd Ed., 1946 Chiropractic Educational Extension Bureau
- Krusen, F., Physical Medicine; 1941 W. B. Saunders Co.
- Clayton, E.R., *Actinotherapy and Diathermy for the Student*; 1939. Ballers, Tindall & Cox

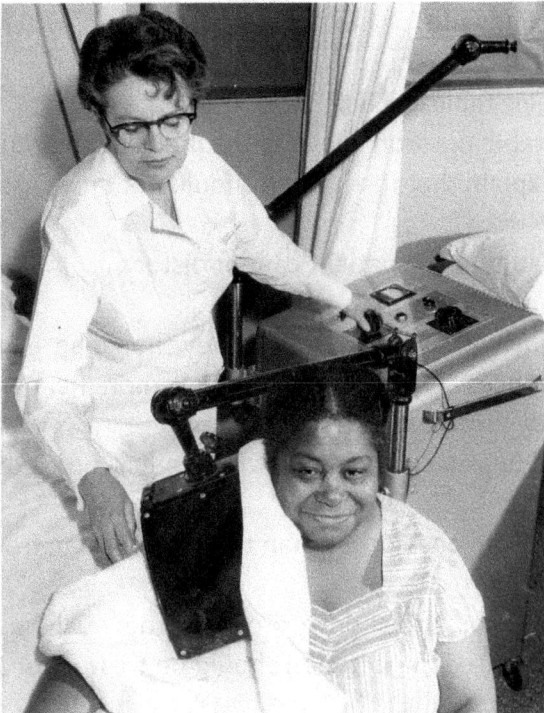

A woman has her arthritic shoulder treated with short wave diathermy.
(Detroit News)

ELECTROTHERAPY

PEMF (Pulsed Electromagnetic Fields)

E

DESCRIPTION

Magnetic fields are generated by electric current running through metal wire coils (called solenoids) or, around a radiant circuit. The mechanism producing the electric current regulated the frequency and the intensity of the magnetic field it creates. This therapy was originally called "low field magnetic stimulation".

There are two categories of PEMF therapy devices:
• Devices that use short radio waves to create a high-frequency, low-intensity electromagnetic field for therapeutic use. This would include short wave diathermy machines used at a low, non-thermal intensity (See **Short Wave Diathermy**).
• Devices that emit pulsed electromagnetic fields using solenoids in contact with the skin. In this case, the devices emit a low-frequency, high intensity field for therapeutic use.

High-frequency devices are more recommended for the treatment of soft tissues, and promote healing, the re-absorption of edema, and the reduction of inflammation. The frequency, measured in megahertz (MHz), can vary from around 18 MHz up to as much as 900 MHz, while the intensity is very low and is usually measured in milliwatts (mW).

Low-frequency devices allow for the treatment of pathologies related to the skeletal system, such as osteoporosis, arthritis, and fractures. They make use of solenoids, and the frequency and intensity are respectively measured in hertz (Hz) and gauss (G).

EQUIPMENT NEEDED
• PEMF generator
• Properly sized pad attachments for the areas treated
• Coil or loop antenna attachment for larger regional application
• Large mat, if full body application is desired

Note: A pulsed short wave diathermy device, with power turned down to below thermal range, will produce PEMF. Magnetic fields are a byproduct of diathermy and can obviate the need for multiple machines.

EFFECTS AND PURPOSE
Clinical studies in this field have shown that such electromagnetic fields are able to regenerate a bio-magnetic field at the cellular level, favoring the intra- and extra-cellular exchange of nutrients and waste. Pulsed magnetic fields have been found to reduce inflammation and pain, enhance biological functionality, accelerate the tissue healing process, and aid in clinical recovery.

INDICATIONS FOR USE
Inflammation, chronic pain, arthritis, fibromyalgia, osteoporosis, fractures, slow wound healing, low back pain and sciatica, post-operative pain and swelling, migraines with aura, depression.

CONTRAINDICATIONS
- Pregnant women
- Children
- Diabetics
- Patients with heart conditions
- Patients with severe arrhythmias
- Epileptics
- Those suffering from tuberculosis, viral diseases (in acute phases), mycoses and acute infections
- Implanted pacemakers
- Patients who use magnetizable prostheses or implants

PRECAUTIONS
Patient should wear cotton or other natural fabric clothing.

ADVANTAGES
- Painless
- Minimal setup

DISADVANTAGES
- Treatment duration for skin contact devices is very long, at least 3-4 hours daily for 45 consecutive days, if using low energy devices.

- Professional equipment is expensive. However, the technology is no mystery and can be self-made using off the shelf components with a little know-how.

INSTRUCTIONS
1. Explain the process to patient.
2. Have patient remove all metal and electronic devices (car keys, cell phone, credit cards with magnetic strip, etc.).
3. Have patient hydrated before and after session.
4. Place patient on a <u>non-metallic</u> table or chair.
5. Position patient in a comfortable position allowing the machine to accurately aim at the treatment site. Explain that the patient should not move around once the treatment begins.
6. Place applicator on target area. Ensure good contact with skin or through thin clothing.
7. Set the intensity and frequency according to therapeutic goals. It should be comfortable for the patient. Most devices offer pre-programmed settings for pain relief, sleep, or stress reduction, which are a good starting point for therapy.
8. Begin therapy with a lower intensity and increase in later sessions as the body adapts. Always record settings for that session.
9. Follow manufacturer's recommendations for treatment duration.

FREQUENCY OF TREATMENT
Daily sessions are considered necessary by the industry

REFERENCES
- Myers, Bryant; *PEMF - The Fifth Element of Health*, 2013 Balboa Press
- Michlovitz, S., *Thermal Agents in Rehabilitation*, 3rd Ed.; 1996 F.A. Davis Co.
- Vadalà, M., Morales-Medina, J. C., Vallelunga, A., Palmieri, B., Laurino, C., & Iannitti, T.; *Pulsed Electromagnetic Field Therapy Effectiveness in Low Back Pain: a Systematic Review of Randomized Controlled Trials.* https://www.elsevier.es/es-revista-porto-biomedical-journal-445-articulo-pulsed-electromagnetic-field-therapy-effectiveness-S2444866416300514
- *Mechanisms and Therapeutic Effectiveness of Pulsed Electromagnetic Field Therapy in Oncology.* (2016). Cancer Med., 5(11), 3128-3139. https://doi.org/10.1002/cam4.861
- Bartolomeo, M. D., Cavani, F., Pellacani, A., Grande, A., Salvatori, R., Chiarini, L., Nocini, R., & Anesi, A; *Pulsed Electro-Magnetic Field (PEMF) Effect on Bone Healing in Animal Models: a Review of its Efficacy Related to Different Type of Damage* (2022). Biology, 11(3). https://doi.org/10.3390/biology11030402

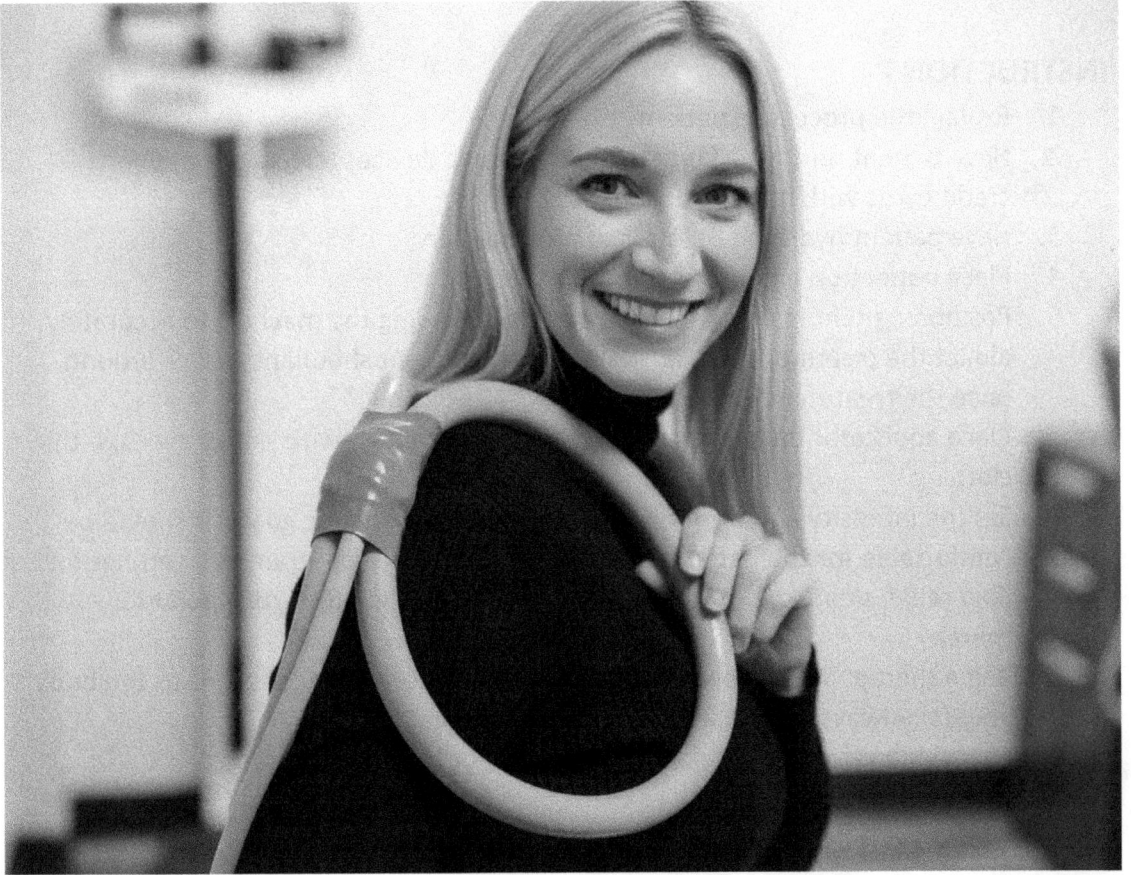

A woman undergoes PEMF therapy with a magnetic coil.

ELECTROTHERAPY

ULTRASOUND DIATHERMY

E

DESCRIPTION

Ultrasound is a type of diathermy that uses sound waves in place of radio waves. They are of such high frequency that they are not perceptible to the human ear, hence the "ultra"—they are beyond sound. The power of the sonic waves delivered to the body are measured in Watts, and are monitored by a meter on the machine.

EQUIPMENT NEEDED

The frequency range allotted for therapeutic ultrasound is 0.8 MHz to 3 MHz. Older units were manufactured at a standard 1 MHz; over time, 3 MHz came to be favored because it is more easily absorbed. However, it does not penetrate as deeply and is better applied to more shallow target tissues (1-2 cm from the skin surface). This makes it more applicable for conditions like tennis elbow and ankle sprains. 1 MHz is preferable for deeper penetration, as larger muscle injuries would demand. Now many companies make dual frequency machines for this reason. Mettler Electronics, Roscoe, and Chattanooga are reputable firms making ultrasound equipment.

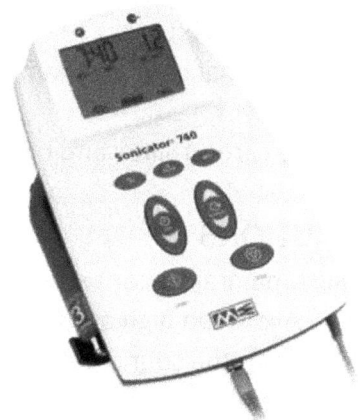

Mettler Sonicator®

EFFECTS AND PURPOSE

As a form of diathermy, ultrasound is a way of delivering therapeutic heat to the tissues. However, not all of its effects can be attributed to its thermal properties. Mechanical and chemical effects are non-thermal, as well as cavitations (vibratory effect causing expansion and compression of gas bubbles).

INDICATIONS FOR USE

- Subacute and chronic inflammation
- Myalgia
- Strains and sprains
- Trigger points
- Joint contractures
- Scarring and fibrosis
- Warts

CONTRAINDICATIONS

- Active bleeding
- Reduced local circulation
- Over anesthetized skin (patient cannot report excessive heating)
- Over gravid uterus
- Over cancerous tumors
- Over the spinal cord post-laminectomy
- Over the eyes
- Over the carotid sinus and cervical ganglia

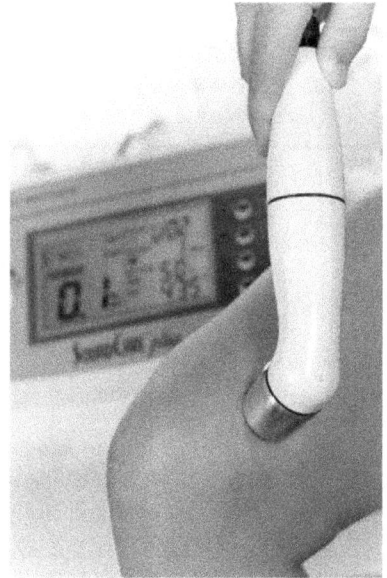

Roscoe Sound Care ultrasound

PRECAUTIONS

You must maintain a consistent energy transfer, or internal burns could result.

1. Avoid too high an intensity.
2. Keep the sound head moving.
3. Maintain even contact.
4. Guard against air bubbles.
5. Avoid bony prominences so ultrasonic energy does not become concentrated in the periosteum
6. Do not hold the powered sound head in the air for more than a few seconds (air does not transmit the waves and the internal crystal in the transducer could shatter or become very hot).

ADVANTAGES

- Short treatment times
- Local effects with few, if any, systemic effects
- Can deliver therapeutic heat deeply to a small area

DISADVANTAGES

- Pressure has to be exerted on the part treated, causing some discomfort in tender tissues
- Dosage difficult to monitor due to little sensation on the part of the patient

INSTRUCTIONS

Superficial conditions or thinner tissues require a lower intensity setting. Painful conditions respond better to moderate intensity settings. Contractions and shortened connective tissue, or thicker tissue, requires higher intensity to achieve a higher temperature within the tissues. As a general rule, the more acute the condition is, the lower the intensity used. The more chronic, the more power used, but <u>patient tolerance is always the final arbiter</u>.

Measure the sound head you are using. The power used is dependent on the size of contact area. A low intensity treatment would be 0.5 Watts per square centimeter; that is, if your sound head was 3 cm diameter, low power would be a setting of 4.5 W (3 x 3 x 0.5). Moderate power is 1-2 W/cm^2 and high power is 2.5-3 W/cm^2 .

Duration of treatments is typically 5-10 minutes per site; 5 minutes for each 25 square inches treated. No therapeutic effects occur in less than 3 minutes, and no additional benefit is gained from more than 10 minutes.

1. Explain procedure to patient.
2. Identify area being treated; sonic waves are very localized, so they must be directed accurately to the site of dysfunction.
3. Position patient for comfort, draping as needed to allow exposure of the target area.
4. Select appropriate frequency setting on the machine.
5. Apply coupling agent (conductive gel) or mineral oil to the target area.
6. Place transducer sound head against the skin and slowly turn up the intensity dial until the proper wattage is reached on the meter.
7. For machines with manual tuning, turn the tuning dial until the light reaches its highest point.
8. Using circular or back-and-forth movements, slide the sound head across the skin, keeping it in firm contact. It should move at the rate of about 4 inches per

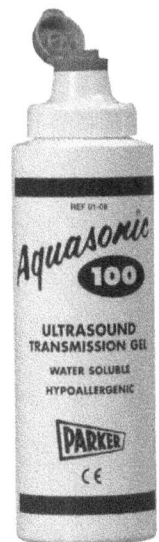

second. Each stroke should overlap, covering half the area of the previous stroke. The sound head <u>must remain parallel to the skin</u> and not be angled.

9. For very small areas, the sound head can be held stationary, but the wattage must be turned down to a minimum to prevent burning.

10. If the sound head has trouble gliding, add more coupler to the skin but do not allow the sound head to rise into the air.

11. After treating for 5-10 minutes per site, turn down the intensity dial, power off the machine, and then remove the applicator/sound head.

12. Clean off the sound head and clean the patient's skin and dry it.

13. Inspect the treated area for any changes and physiological response.

FREQUENCY OF TREATMENT
Initially daily in acute injury, less often in subacute and chronic cases.

REFERENCES
- Michlovitz, S., *Thermal Agents in Rehabilitation*, 3rd Ed.; 1996 F.A. Davis Co.
- Johnson, A.C., *Principles and Practice of Drugless Therapeutics*; 3rd Ed., 1946 Chiropractic Educational Extension Bureau
- Krusen, F., Physical Medicine; 1941 W. B. Saunders Co.
- Handbook of Physical Medicine; 1945 American Medical Association

ELECTROTHERAPY

PHONOPHORESIS

E

DESCRIPTION
The use of ultrasound diathermy to ionically transfer medicinal substances to the body by driving them into the tissues using high frequency sound waves.

EQUIPMENT NEEDED
Any of the conventionally available ultrasound devices can be used for phonophoresis. The previously stated advantage over other ionization using galvanic current is that polarity is not an issue. It is more a matter of ensuring that the ionic solution is well absorbed from the driving force of the sonic waves, because of the natural acoustic impedance of the flesh.

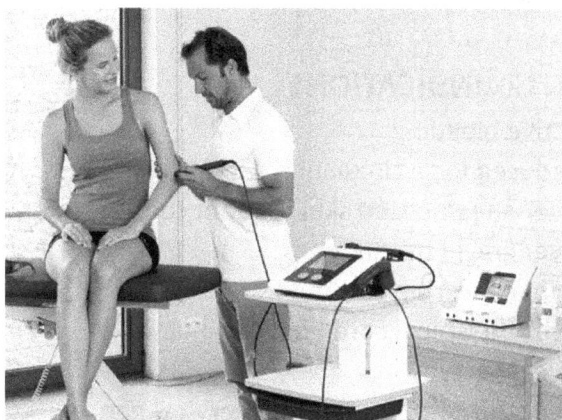
Fizyomed® ultrasound

Direct method
One can apply the ion solution to the skin before proceeding, or prepare a combined medication/conductive gel. If mixing the medicated solution with a coupling agent as is used in ultrasound, the coupling agent should be a good water-based gel. A petrolatum-type coupler is not applicable. Any undissolved solid ingredients must be finely dispersed in the vehicle. The aqueous coupler serves the dual purpose of containing the medicinal substances and preventing air bubbles from arising between the transducer and the patient's skin, thus reducing absorption of the medication. It must provide good ultrasonic energy conduction, be homogeneous, smooth and not gritty. It must also have relatively low viscosity for easier application and movement of the transducer head.

Indirect method

One can mix the ion solution in a basin of water, bathe the affected body part in the water, and submerge the transducer head in the water to create indirect phonophoresis. Place the sound head parallel to the target area and one inch away. The ultrasonic energy will cause the solution to permeate the water and penetrate the skin. Because the water is the coupling agent, and there are no air gaps, the ultrasound will encounter no impedance.

EFFECTS AND PURPOSE

All the benefits of ultrasound therapy with the added benefit of ionic medication.

INDICATIONS FOR USE

All conditions that would benefit from ultrasound, as well as conditions listed in the protocols list in the **Ionization** section.

CONTRAINDICATIONS

- Active bleeding
- Reduced local circulation
- Over anesthetized skin (patient cannot report excessive heating)
- Over gravid uterus
- Over cancerous tumors
- Over the spinal cord post-laminectomy
- Over the eyes
- Over the carotid sinus and cervical ganglia

PRECAUTIONS

You must maintain a consistent energy transfer, or internal burns could result.

1. Avoid too high an intensity.
2. Keep the sound head moving.
3. Maintain even contact.
4. Guard against air bubbles.
5. Avoid bony prominences so ultrasonic energy does not become concentrated in the periosteum
6. Do not hold the powered sound head in the air for more than a few seconds (air does not transmit the waves and the internal crystal in the transducer could shatter or become very hot).

ADVANTAGES

- Short treatment times
- Can deliver biochemical changes without using injection or oral agents
- Ion solution materials can be purchased in bulk for little cost

DISADVANTAGES

Equipment can be moderately expensive

INSTRUCTIONS

Direct method

1. Explain procedure to patient.
2. Position patient for comfort, draping as needed to allow exposure of the target area.
3. Identify area being treated; sonic waves are very localized, so they must be directed accurately to the site of dysfunction.
4. Prepare ion solution according to the chart in the Ionization section.
5. Apply to the target area on the skin first, then apply coupling gel.
6. Select appropriate frequency setting on the machine.
7. Apply coupling agent (conductive gel) to the target area. Do not use mineral oil in this application.
8. Place transducer sound head against the skin and slowly turn up the intensity dial until the proper wattage is reached on the meter.
9. For machines with manual tuning, turn the tuning dial until the light reaches its highest point.
10. Using circular or back-and-forth movements, slide the sound head across the skin, keeping it in firm contact. It should move at the rate of about 4 inches per second. Each stroke should overlap, covering half the area of the previous stroke. The sound head must remain parallel to the skin and not be angled.
11. For very small areas, the sound head can be held stationary, but the wattage must be turned down to a minimum to prevent burning.
12. If the sound head has trouble gliding, add more coupler to the skin but do not allow the sound head to rise into the air.
13. After treating for 5-10 minutes per site, turn down the intensity dial, power off the machine, and then remove the applicator/sound head.
14. Clean off the sound head and clean the patient's skin and dry it.
15. Inspect the treated area for any changes and physiological response.

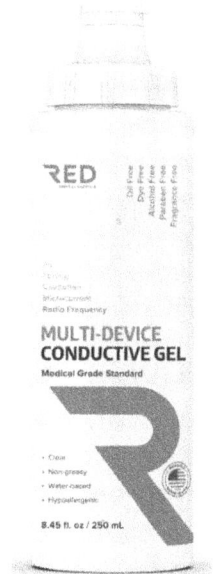

Red Medical Supplies makes an excellent aqueous gel.

Indirect method
1. Explain procedure to the patient.
2. Mix the ion solution in a basin of water,
3. Bathe the affected body part in the water
4. Submerge the transducer head in the water to create indirect phonophoresis.
5. Place the sound head parallel to the target area and one inch away.
6. The ultrasonic energy will cause the solution to permeate the water and penetrate the skin. Because the water is the coupling agent, and there are no air gaps, the ultrasound will encounter no impedance.
7. Slowly turn up the intensity dial until the proper wattage is reached on the meter.
8. For machines with manual tuning, turn the tuning dial until the light reaches its highest point.
9. Treat for 5-10 minutes.
10. Turn down the intensity dial, power off the machine, and remove the transducer.
11. Dry the patient and clean the transducer head.

FREQUENCY OF TREATMENT
Initially daily in acute injury, less often in subacute and chronic cases.

REFERENCES
- Michlovitz, S., *Thermal Agents in Rehabilitation*, 3rd Ed.; 1996 F.A. Davis Co.
- Hayes, K., *Manual for Physical Agents;* 4th Ed., 1984 Appleton & Lange
- Krusen, F., Physical Medicine; 1941 W. B. Saunders Co.

ELECTROTHERAPY

Motor Point Stimulation

E

DESCRIPTION

Motor points are spots on the skin where a nerve branches out in a muscle (motor end plate) and the nerve is closest to the skin surface. They will trigger a contraction of that muscle with a minimal amount of electrical stimulation. Electrical stimulation of these points can also relax the muscle. The points are often located at the junction of the upper and middle third of the belly of the muscle.

There are two possibilities for electrical stimulation of motor points[4]:

1. **Monophasic** (Unipolar) stimulation
2. **Biphasic** (Bipolar) stimulation

Monophasic stimulation tends to be somewhat painful for motor point stimulation, and is not generally used (although it can be effective if there is no biphasic equipment available). Of the biphasic currents, the faradic is the stronger and more applicable current for achieving motor point response.

EQUIPMENT NEEDED

As has been discussed previously in this book, faradic current has been largely abandoned by conventional physiotherapy in the USA to the extent that electrotherapy equipment with multiple settings often do not include faradic stimulation. However, Mettler Electronics makes a number of devices specifically for neuromuscular stimulation. New Life Care in India makes a faradic instrument. A small unit with both faradic and galvanic (monophasic) settings is made by Acco™.

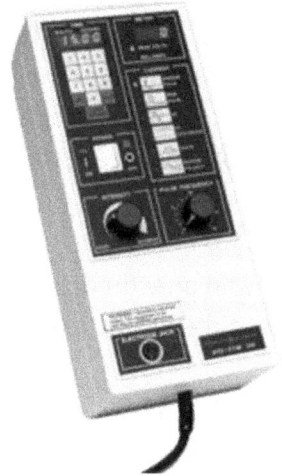

The Mettler **Sys*Stim 206** is a versatile device that can perform motor point stimulation as well as other therapies.

---

[4] Acupuncture can also be used.

EFFECTS AND PURPOSE

Motor point stimulation is a way to provide exercise to muscles that cannot contract voluntarily. It can help maintain nutrition and blood flow in the denervated muscle, and lessen denervation atrophy. In innervated muscles, it strengthens them, increases peripheral blood flow, increases mobility, and prevents fibrosis.

Most motor points are also acupuncture points. One can achieve acupuncture effects from electrical stimulation of the points without penetrating the skin, while at the same time creating motor point effects on the musculature. If using bipolar stimulation, two acupuncture points can be stimulated at once; and, if both are located at motor end-points, excite a muscle response also.

INDICATIONS FOR USE
- Nerve injuries
- Tendon transplants
- Denervated/atrophied muscles
- Poor mobility
- To prevent fibrotic changes

CONTRAINDICATIONS
- Do not apply over the chest or heart region in patients with pacemakers
- Do not apply over open wounds, skin infections
- Do not apply over areas with cancerous tumors.

PRECAUTIONS
- Avoid anesthetic skin areas if possible (if necessary, use lower intensity)
- Avoid extreme edema

ADVANTAGES
- The current intensity required to produce muscle contraction is small, compared to any other area on the muscle belly
- The optimum contraction of each muscle can be obtained

DISADVANTAGES
- Some mild sensory irritation or discomfort
- Induced fatigue
- Control of current dosage is sometimes challenging

INSTRUCTIONS

1. Explain the procedure to the patient. Describe the sensations likely to be felt.
2. Check the skin condition and also the sensory perception at the chosen treatment site.
3. If the skin at the site is oily or has cosmetics on it, wash with soap and water before commencing treatment. If the skin is cold, warm it first to increase circulation and perspiration, which help conductivity of the electricity.
4. Position patient so that you have complete access to the limb under treatment. The limb should be in a mostly extended position in order to produce a contraction, if the goal is to strengthen. An impaired limb will fall back during the rest cycle of the stimulation, so precautions should be taken to prevent injury.
5. Place indifferent (dispersive) electrode against the body some distance from the treatment site but on the same side of the body (ipsilaterally). It should be secured either by body weight or by strap or adhesive contact.
6. Connect cable from the indifferent electrode to the device.
7. Connect the cable from a pencil electrode with an interruptor switch to the device. This is the active electrode.
8. If using a monophasic current[5], the <u>active electrode should be connected to the negative pole</u>. If using a biphasic current, the polarity is irrelevant.
9. Set stimulator to appropriate setting for the condition. A frequency of at least 30 Hz is necessary for a smooth muscle contraction. Higher frequencies than 30 Hz are more comfortable but also fatiguing.
10. Innervated muscles require a fast rise time of 200-300 microseconds.
11. Denervated muscles require a longer duration stimulation. A rise time of 100 milliseconds is typical.
12. Check motor point charts and place the active electrode in the approximate spot.
13. Press firmly and close the switch. Turn intensity dial up from zero until you see a contraction begin.
14. Observe the strength of the contraction. Move the electrode around to find the place of maximum response. That will be the motor point. The stimulation there will be more comfortable to the patient because of the decreased resistance at the point.
15. If at any point the treatment is interrupted, return the intensity to zero and re-start the process.

---

[5] Monophasic stimulation can often cause contractions in adjacent muscles, distracting from the target muscle. For this reason, biphasic currents have come to be used for this purpose, which are less likely to wander.

16. For strengthening: Increase intensity level until you have a strong contraction (but not painful). By depressing the switch, create 20-25 contractions. The stronger the intensity, the fewer are needed.
17. For muscle re-education: Apply only moderate contractions. Intermittently produce 3-10 contractions at the outset, gradually increasing in sequential sessions to 30-40.
18. Always set intensity back to zero before breaking contact with the patient's skin.

FREQUENCY OF TREATMENT

Denervated muscles are typically stimulated 3 times daily with at least 10 minutes rest between sessions.

Innervated muscles can be treated once or twice a week.

REFERENCES

- Hayes, K., *Manual for Physical Agents;* 4th Ed., 1984 Appleton & Lange
- Johnson, A.C., *Principles and Practice of Drugless Therapeutics*; 3rd Ed., 1946 Chiropractic Educational Extension Bureau
- Krusen, F., Physical Medicine; 1941 W. B. Saunders Co.
- Handbook of Physical Medicine; 1945 American Medical Association
- Morse, F., *Low Volt Currents of Physiotherapy*; 1925 General X-Ray Co.

MOTOR POINTS

(after Morse)

UPPER EXTREMITIES

ANTERIOR

POSTERIOR

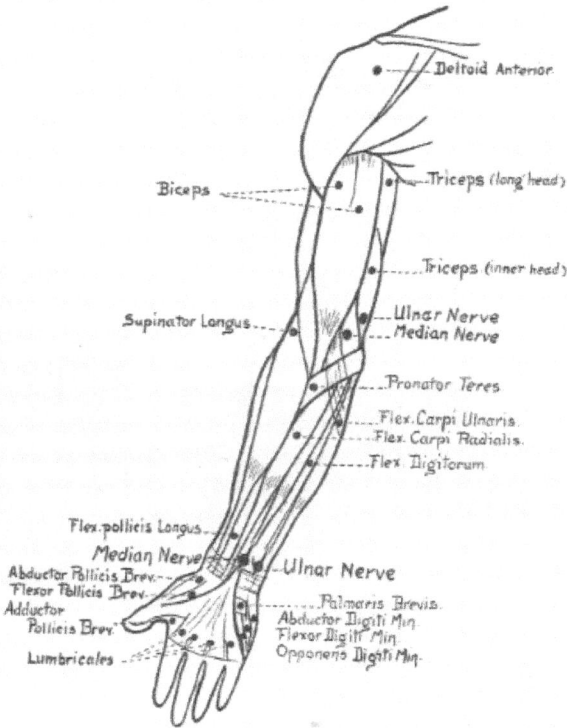

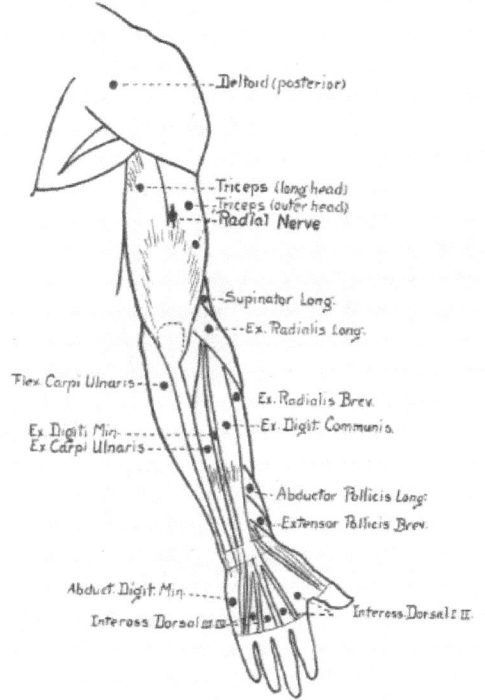

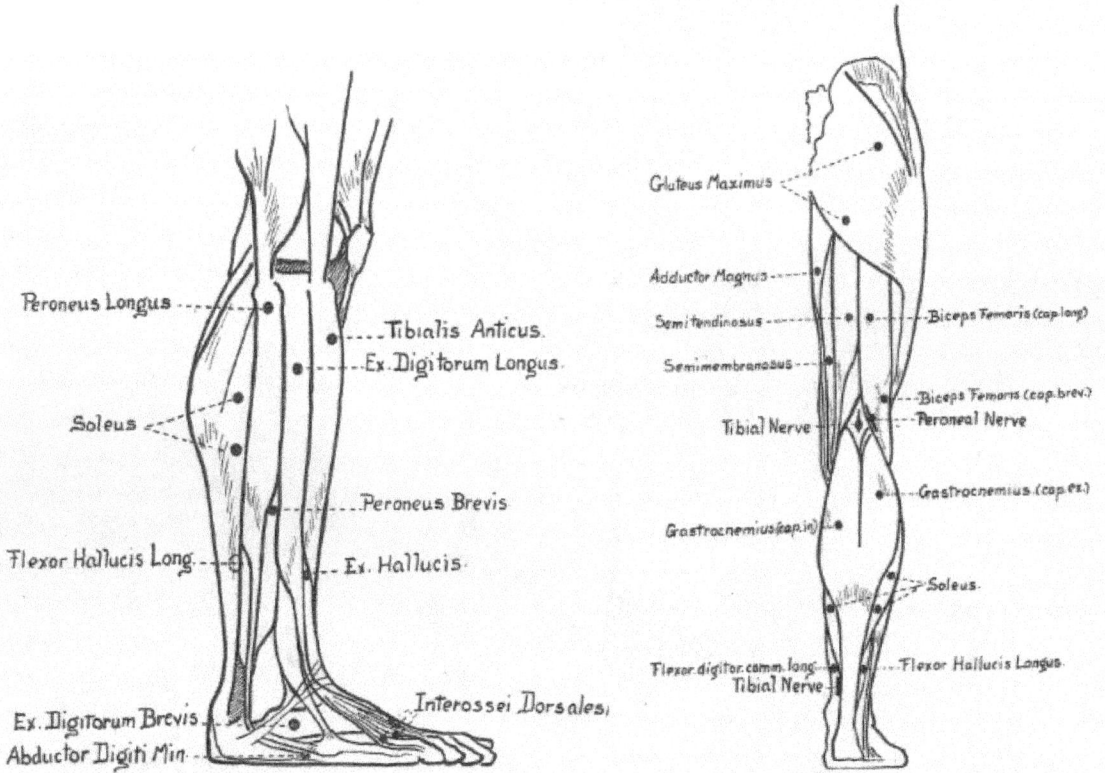

Peroneus Longus

Tibialis Anticus.

Ex. Digitorum Longus.

Soleus

Peroneus Brevis

Flexor Hallucis Long.

Ex. Hallucis.

Ex. Digitorum Brevis.

Abductor Digiti Min.

Interossei Dorsales,

Gluteus Maximus

Adductor Magnus

Semitendinosus

Biceps Femoris (cap.long)

Semimembranosus

Biceps Femoris (cap.brev.)

Tibial Nerve

Peroneal Nerve

Gastrocnemius (cap.ex.)

Gastrocnemius(cap.in)

Soleus.

Flexor digitor. comm. long.
Tibial Nerve

Flexor Hallucis Longus.

ANTERIOR

POSTERIOR

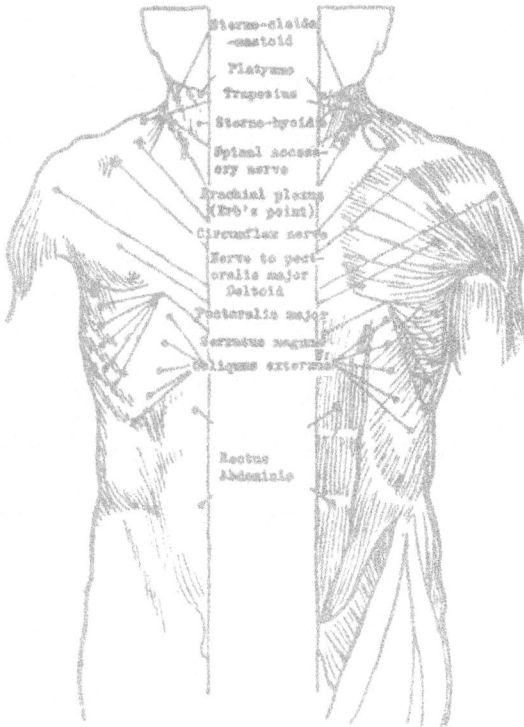
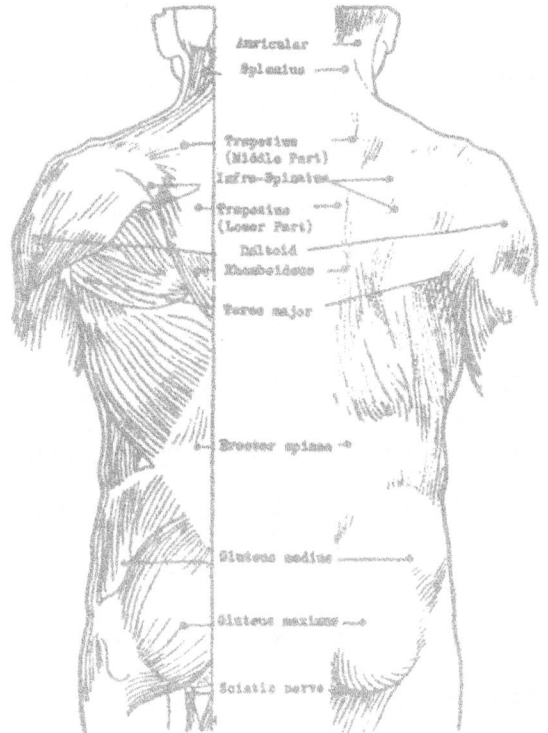

Sterno-cleido-mastoid
Platysma
Trapezius
Sterno-hyoid
Spinal accessory nerve
Brachial plexus (Erb's point)
Circumflex nerve
Nerve to pectoralis major
Deltoid
Pectoralis major
Serratus magnus
Obliquus externus
Rectus Abdominis

Auricular
Splenius
Trapezius (Middle Part)
Infra-Spinatus
Trapezius (Lower Part)
Deltoid
Rhomboideus
Teres major
Erector spinae
Gluteus medius
Gluteus maximus
Sciatic nerve

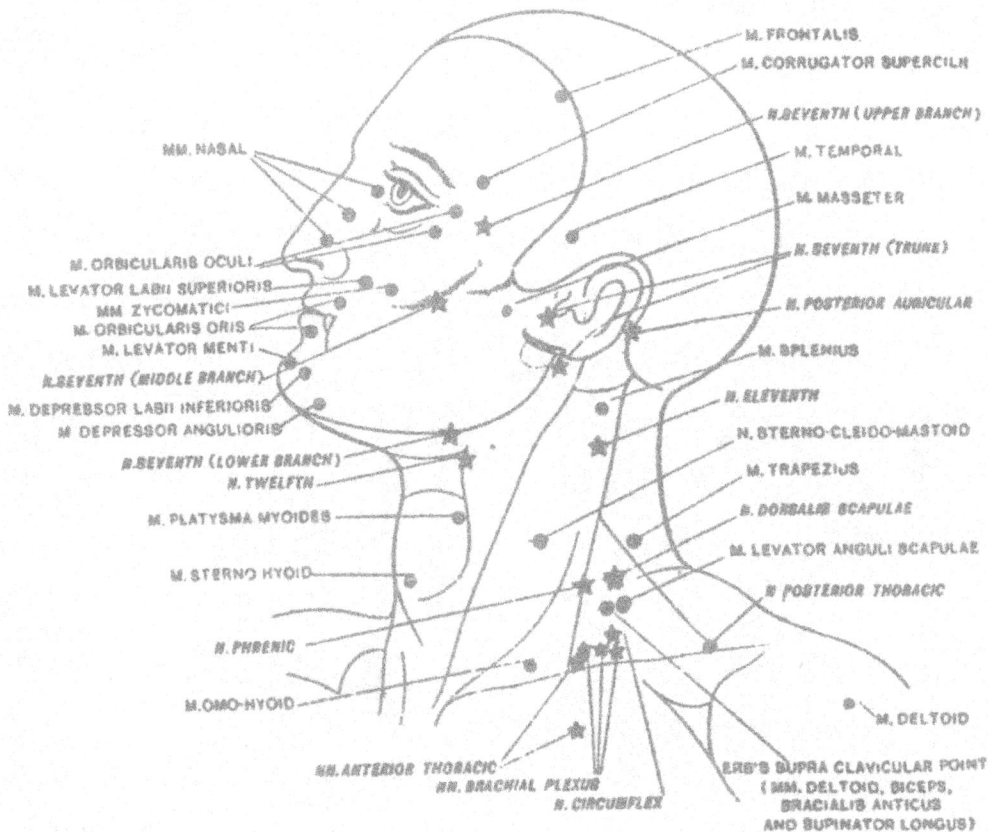

M. FRONTALIS
M. CORRUGATOR SUPERCILII
N. SEVENTH (UPPER BRANCH)
M. TEMPORAL
M. MASSETER
N. SEVENTH (TRUNK)
N. POSTERIOR AURICULAR
M. SPLENIUS
N. ELEVENTH
N. STERNO-CLEIDO-MASTOID
M. TRAPEZIUS
B. DORSALIS SCAPULAE
M. LEVATOR ANGULI SCAPULAE
N. POSTERIOR THORACIC
M. DELTOID

MM. NASAL

M. ORBICULARIS OCULI
M. LEVATOR LABII SUPERIORIS
MM. ZYCOMATICI
M. ORBICULARIS ORIS
M. LEVATOR MENTI
N. SEVENTH (MIDDLE BRANCH)
M. DEPRESSOR LABII INFERIORIS
M. DEPRESSOR ANGULIORIS
N. SEVENTH (LOWER BRANCH)
N. TWELFTH
M. PLATYSMA MYOIDES
M. STERNO HYOID
N. PHRENIC
M. OMO-HYOID

NN. ANTERIOR THORACIC
NN. BRACHIAL PLEXUS
N. CIRCUMFLEX

ERB'S SUPRA CLAVICULAR POINT
(MM. DELTOID, BICEPS,
BRACIALIS ANTICUS
AND SUPINATOR LONGUS)

7

MECHANICAL VIBRATION

VIBROTHERAPY or "RHYTHMOTHERAPY"

DESCRIPTION

The use of mechanical devices that vibrate and/or make percussive impact to the myofascial tissues for therapeutic effect. The term "Rhythmotherapy" is now archaic, but is mentioned because it is enshrined in law as one of the modalities originally designated for use by Doctors of Naturopathy. It was even referred to at one time as "Sysmotherapy".

Mechanical vibration (oscillation) and mechanical percussion are the two modes of Vibrotherapy and can sometimes be delivered by the same equipment.

EQUIPMENT NEEDED

An oscillator (British: *Gyrator*)has an internal offset cam that produces vibration; a percussor makes linear in-and-out thrusts.

Turonic massager/ percussor has 5 adjustable speeds and a variety of heads for versatile use.

There are historically various attachments for applying to different body parts.

- A ball head is used for large muscles
- A flat head for chest and back muscles
- A fork head for shoulders, neck, and spinal column
- A cone head for small muscles in hands and feet, and for trigger points
- A steel cylinder head for deep oil massage

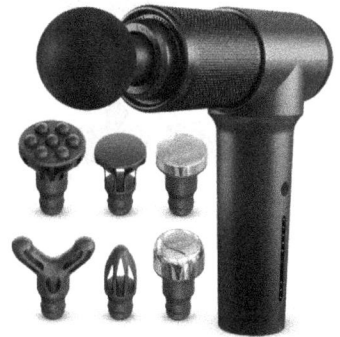

For many years, the company G5 (General Physiotherapy, Inc.)has been the pre-eminent producer of such physiotherapy devices in North America. They combine oscillation and percussion in one unit. However, there are other simpler and more moderately priced apparatus on the market.

EFFECTS AND PURPOSE

Vibration (oscillation) increases lymphatic drainage and blood circulation, thus detoxifying the tissues and bringing nutrition to them, respectively. Percussion tonifies the muscles (increases tone) and increases blood circulation. It is used most often on the shoulders, arms, and back.

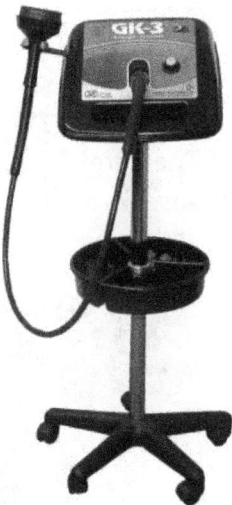

The GK-3 percussor has a variable speed control, from 15-60 pulses per second.

INDICATIONS FOR USE

- •Soft tissue pain
- •Restricted range of motion
- •Paresthesia
- •Repetitive strain injuries
- •Prevent delayed onset muscle soreness
- •Increase flexibility
- •Sprains
- •Edema
- •Tension headaches
- •Anxiety
- •Bronchial conditions and airway clearance (percussion): Bronchiectasis, COPD, Cystic Fibrosis,

CONTRAINDICATIONS

- •Bleeding disorder
- •Local bruising
- •Underlying tumors
- •Percussive stimulation should not be used in radiculopathy

PRECAUTIONS

- Inspect the area(s) being treated to spot any anomalies before beginning.
- Deep tissue stimulation should always be done to tolerance.

ADVANTAGES

- Does not tire the therapist like manual massage
- Produces a deeper, more powerful action than by hands
- Shorter treatment time allows more patients to be seen

DISADVANTAGES

The more sophisticated the device, the more expensive.

INSTRUCTIONS

For all types of devices, <u>high speed</u> setting is recommended for general relaxation, relaxing specific muscles groups and relieving spasm, reducing trigger points, stimulating blood circulation, and creating analgesia to relieve pain. <u>Medium speed</u> settings are recommended for all of the same, except when a deeper effect is desired. <u>Low speed</u> settings are used for toning muscles that are weak, for applying to sensitive areas, for postural drainage in pulmonary conditions, and for use on children and the elderly.

1. Explain procedure to patient before starting.
2. Choose action setting on the device.
3. Place on hand on the body area being treated, palpating the tissues ahead of the applicator.
4. Support and move the tissues into a more accessible position with the guiding hand if needed as you move the head of the vibrator with the other hand.
5. Move the applicator slowly at all times.
6. Always work distal to proximal, in the direction of venous and lymphatic flow.

Treatment durations:

- General relaxation: 3-5 minutes
- Relaxation of specific muscles: 2-5 minutes
- Localized therapy: 5 minutes or less; less time for acute, more for chronic cases
- Reducing trigger points: 2-6 <u>seconds</u>
- Postural drainage: 5 minutes or less per treated area, less for an acute episode

FREQUENCY OF TREATMENT

Determined by case

REFERENCES

- Lake, T. T., *Treatment By Neuropathy and The Encyclopedia of Manipulative Therapeutics;* 1946
- Eberhart, N.M., *A Brief Physiotherapy Manual,* 1928 New Medicine Pub. Co.
- Brown, B.H., *Vibratory Technique,* 2nd Edition, 1914 Vibratory Pub. Co.,Chicago
- Snow, A., *Mechanical Vibration And Its Therapeutic Application,* 1904 Scientific Authors' Pub. Co.

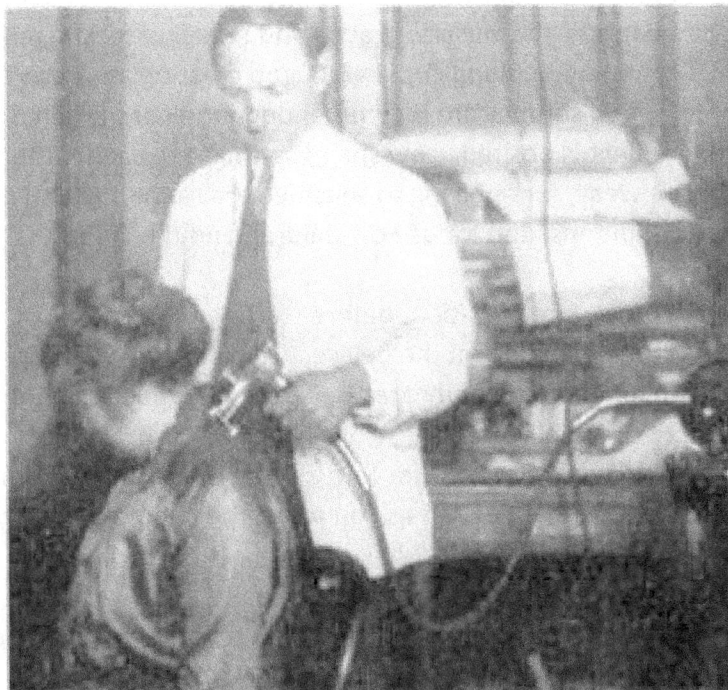

Joe Shelby Riley, ND using an electric percussor

8

MECHANOTHERAPY

MASSOTHERAPY / MYOTHERAPY

DESCRIPTION

Massotherapy is the traditional term for medically oriented therapeutic massage; mechanical manipulation of skin, connective tissue and muscles for the purpose of enhancing health. It is the rubbing or kneading of the body's soft tissues, commonly applied with hands, fingers, elbows, knees, forearms, feet, or a device. Massotherapy has physiological and psychological benefits.

M

Various specialized technics fall under this heading, such as Myotherapy and its precursors Neuromuscular Technique, and Trigger Point Therapy. There are also maneuvers such as Proprioceptive Neuromuscular Facilitation (PNF), Myofascial Release, etc. Myotherapy will be discussed shortly.

The different technics within conventional Ling Method (Swedish Movement) massotherapy are as follows:

> • <u>Stroking</u> (*Effleurage*), a light, continuous movement stroking movement applied with the fingers and palms over the skin in a slow, rhythmic motion. Very little pressure is applied; the skin is lightly touched, creating a relaxing effect. The pads of the fingers are used over small surfaces and the palms are used over larger surfaces. The wrist and fingertips are lightly curved to conform to the area being massaged, and just the pads of the fingers (or the surface of the palms) make contact.

• Kneading (*Petrissage*), a pulling and kneading movement where the flesh is grasped between the operator's palms and the fingers. As the tissues are raised from their underlying structures, they are rolled, squeezed, or pinched with a light but firm pressure. Used primarily on the shoulders and back in clinical practice, it is invigorating and increases circulation in the deeper myofascial tissues. Kneading movements are light but firm. Pulling is used often on the arms. The fingers of both hands grasp the arm and apply a kneading movement that separates the fibers and stretches the tissues.

• Percussion (*Tapotement*), a technic that uses slapping, tapping, or hacking (chopping motions with the edge of the hand). Slapping uses a flexible wrist, permitting the palms to come into contact with the patient's skin in a series of light but firm, rapid slapping movements. Tapping involves bringing flexed fingers down in rapid succession to stimulate a small area. Hacking uses the ulnar edge of the hands to alternately percuss the flesh. Wrists and fingers have to be supple in order to do this with any coordination. Percussion movements tonify the muscles (increase tone) and increase blood circulation. They are used most often on the shoulders, arms, and back.

• Vibration, a stimulating technic that greatly increases superficial and deep circulation. It is traditionally performed by rapid contractions of the operator's arms while the fingertips are planted firmly on the area being treated. While it can be performed manually, it can also be accomplished by mechanical means with an electric or mechanical vibrator. Care must be taken when using vibration not to aggravate any present nerve root irritation. Vibratory technic, manual or mechanical, should best not be used where there is radiculopathy.

• Friction, a technic that penetrates deeper tissues and used mainly on the arms and legs. Variations include rubbing, rolling, wringing, and chucking movements. Friction technic has the operator's fingers or palms maintaining pressure on the skin while the skin is being moved over the underlying structures.

Myotherapy

Myotherapy is an outgrowth of Trigger Point Therapy, a manual technic often taught in massotherapy schools, which became well established for effective pain relief. Trigger points are palpable nodules in the muscle or connective tissue, tender when pressed, and found where there are stress patterns, localized spasm, or muscle damage. They are essentially the same as what has been called *ah shi* points in acupuncture for many centuries.

The theory is that normal muscle tone is lost due to injury or prolonged tension. The changed muscle tone can change the positions of the bones, causing spinal subluxations, joint and postural distortions, etc. A trigger point eventually forms in the muscle, which sends a bombardment of impulses into the local area, producing vasoconstriction and resultant ischemia. Since muscle tone is controlled by the sympathetic nervous system, it is not under conscious control and therefore is resistant to self-correction. Pressure applied in the right way to these points will release the "trigger" and the hypertonicity of the muscle.

The Nimmo Receptor-Tonus Method, also known as Nimmo Technic, was developed by Raymond Nimmo, D.C., and was probably the first method (after acupuncture) to center on the principle of treating what came to be called "trigger points". He evolved the method over a 30-year period and began lecturing on it in 1957. Most Chiropractic colleges teach courses in Nimmo Technic. It can relieve pain immediately. Wooden "T- Bars" with rubber tips are held by the operator and used to reach between ribs and transverse processes in order to eliminate trigger points.

Naturopathic doctors often specialize in an offshoot of Nimmo Technic called Neuromuscular Technique, originated by British Naturopath Dr. Stanley Leif. Janet Travell, M.D. called her version of the method Myotherapy, and expanded it to actually injecting the trigger points with local anesthetics, which likewise was borrowed from Neural Therapy, which she studied in Germany. Contemporary myotherapy includes myofascial stretching, corrective exercises, and some deep tissue massage as well.

EQUIPMENT NEEDED
The T-bar is probably the most valuable tool for applying myotherapy, or at least the first that should be acquired.

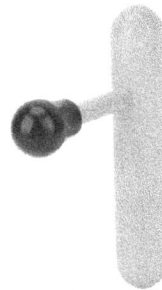

EFFECTS AND PURPOSE

The physiological effects of massage are well documented and voluminous, and will only be summarized here. Properly performed, massotherapy increases blood perfusion in areas treated and increases venous return, resulting in faster transit back to the heart and therefore assist oxygenation of the blood and heightened nutrition to the tissues. In addition, it expels waste products from the muscles and connective tissue, increases lymphatic drainage, and thus aids in a primary naturopathic concept—detoxification of the body.

The mechanisms of myotherapy, on the other hand, are more complicated and controversial. The phenomenon of the trigger point has spawned several theories as to its physiology, and there is as yet no definitive explanation.

INDICATIONS FOR USE
- Soft tissue pain
- Restricted range of motion
- Paresthesia
- Repetitive strain injuries
- Sprains
- Tension headaches

CONTRAINDICATIONS
- Bleeding disorder
- Local bruising
- Underlying tumors
- No massage over gravid uterus or in the first three days of menstruation
- Not advisable over varicose veins

PRECAUTIONS
- Inspect the area(s) being treated to spot any anomalies before beginning.
- Deep tissue stimulation should always be done to tolerance.

ADVANTAGES
- Can be performed almost anywhere
- Requires no special equipment

DISADVANTAGES
- Fatiguing—amount performed will be dependent on physical endurance of the operator.

INSTRUCTIONS
Whether using a massage tool like the T-bar or simply the thumbs, the technic is simple:

1. Find the tender trigger point by palpation.
2. Make continuous deep pressure until the patient's tolerance is reached.
3. Instruct the patient to tell you when the pain starts to fade. When it does, advise that you are going to increase the pressure until a new tolerance level is reached. Once that is accomplished, hold the pressure steady for another 7-15 seconds.
4. When the pain subsides again, repeat the process (usually two or three cycles are performed).
5. Then very gradually begin to release the pressure in a small, circular pattern of movement. This prevents a rebound reflex spasm of the muscle.
6. Finish up with a "milking"of the local muscles by stretching or stroking in the direction of the muscle fibers. It is a somewhat painful procedure but produces dramatic results.

Trigger Point stimulation can be accomplished with other modalities as well. **Ultrasound, low voltage electrical stimulation, infrared**, and cold **lasers** can be applied to the trigger points.

FREQUENCY OF TREATMENT
Because some recovery time is needed, no more than twice a week at most.

REFERENCES
- Finando, D., *Trigger Point Therapy for Myofascial Pain: The Practice of Informed Touch;* 2005 Healing Arts Press
- Prudden, B., *Pain Erasure;* 2002 M. Evans & Co.
- Tappan, F., *Massage Techniques, A Case Method Approach*; 1961 Macmillan Co.

MECHANOTHERAPY

REFLEX or ZONE THERAPY

DESCRIPTION

Zone Therapy, as it was originally called, and Reflexology, as it came to be known, is the practice of manually massaging, kneading, or pushing on areas of the feet, hands, and sometimes the ears, in order to exert an influence on other parts of the body through a reflexive action. The goal is to engender a beneficial effect on those distant parts by way of this reflexive action. It has been a therapy recognized in Naturopathy since the 1920s.

The American Reflexology Certification Board (ARCB) defines Reflexology as "the application of specific pressure using the practitioner's hand, thumb, and fingers to reflex maps resembling the human body, primarily located on the feet and hands. This practice is believed to promote relaxation and support the body's natural functions".

EQUIPMENT NEEDED

Just the hands and fingers, although small cudgels are sometimes used to better stimulate small points (seen at right).

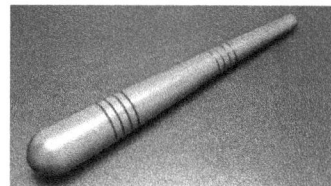

EFFECTS AND PURPOSE

Although there is no consensus as to the exact mechanism or mechanisms by which reflexology works (and therefore has left it open to much criticism as quackery), it has been subjected to medical scrutiny in recent years and found effective for a variety of conditions. This is not unlike Acupuncture.

Zone Therapy was first expounded in the U.S.A. in 1913 by Dr. William H. Fitzgerald, an otolaryngologist, and Dr. Edwin F. Bowers. It is believed that Fitzgerald was first influenced by Cherokee and other Native American tribal methods in his discoveries. Fitzgerald was the first to make the claim that applying pressure to certain areas would have an anesthetic effect on a distant area. In many cases, it not only relieved pain but also eradicated the underlying cause of the pain. He realized that the body is divided into ten longitudinal sections, which he referred to as "zones". With five zones on each side of the midline of the body, each one begins at the crown and runs vertically down to the fingertips and toes. In order to prove the existence of these zones, Dr. Fitzgerald applied rubber bands, clamps, and other probes to apply pressure to these areas to produce anesthesia in specific parts of the related zones.

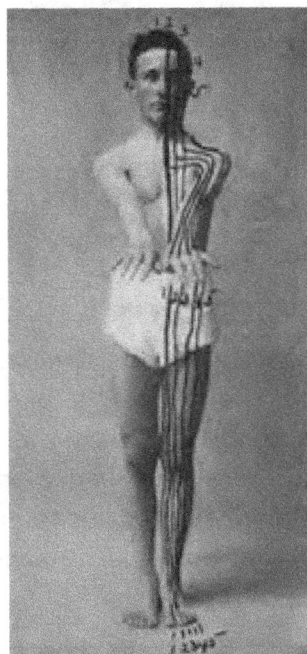

Joe Shelby Riley, DO, ND also studied under Fitzgerald and went on to become the most prominent naturopath teaching Zone Therapy. He further developed Fitzgerald and Bowers' work, and trained many naturopaths to use the therapy (including one of the author's instructors). One student was an osteopathic nurse and physiotherapist named Eunice D. Ingham, who began using the term Reflexology to describe the therapy after training with Riley in the 1930s, and which is now more popularly known. She concentrated on the foot, mapped out more precise locations of the various reflex points, and is considered the "mother" of Reflexology. Her Ingham Method of Reflexology is the most widely known, although there are other more recently developed variations. Hand Reflexology, although used originally by Fitzgerald and Riley, is now increasing in use, as well as ear Reflexology, which likely has been due to the influence of Acupuncture.

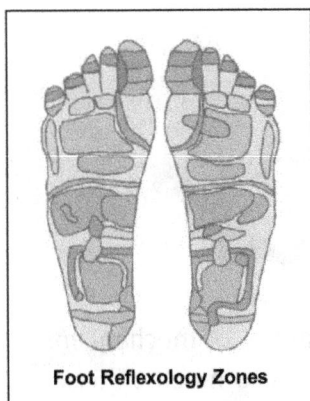

Foot Reflexology Zones

INDICATIONS FOR USE
Pain and functional disorders

CONTRAINDICATIONS
- Bleeding disorder
- Local bruising
- Underlying tumors

PRECAUTIONS
Keep aseptic technique in mind when working on people's feet and hands.

ADVANTAGES
- Can apply anywhere
- Costs next to nothing

DISADVANTAGES
- As with other manual methods, hand fatigue and wear and tear on the joints to a degree is unavoidable.
- The public associates Reflexology with other practitioners rather than naturopaths.

INSTRUCTIONS
For Zone Therapy:
1. Locate the longitudinal zone line running through the site of the ailment by use of the chart at right.
2. Pain in the knee, for example, may be treated by pressure on the corresponding surface on the elbow of the same side.
3. If the pain exists, say, in the left eye or above it, trace the 3rd zone to the middle finger and the third toe.

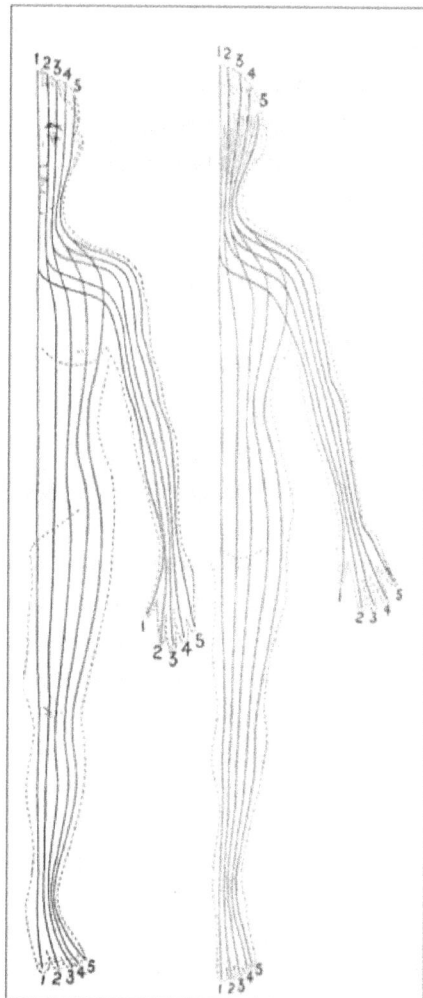

4. Treatment is made by applying pressure over the first joint of the third toe, or the corresponding joint of the middle finger on that side, and any tender or tight spots found anywhere along that zone.
5. Pressure is maintained for 30 seconds to 4 minutes, or even 10 minutes if needed, depending on the reaction of the patient. The pressure can be made with the thumb and fingernails, or a metal comb having ten teeth to the inch. They can also be treated with the steady pressure of a spring clothespin or a rubber band.
6. Pressure can be exerted over any firm bony surface along the path of that zone.
7. Nervous headaches can be relieved by pressure on the roof of the mouth, behind the front incisors.

INSTRUCTIONS
For Reflexology:
A general foot reflexology session involves a foot treatment for about 40 to 45 minutes. It is done with the hand and sometimes a probe or a simple pencil eraser to apply pressure. Use a table or chair adjusted to the right elevation so that you do not strain. Keep fingernails trimmed short. Have a supply of towels handy.

1. Wash and sanitize the feet with warm water infused with Epsom salt. Dry thoroughly.
2. Observe the feet for cuts, bruises, or anomalies.
3. Begin with gentle effleurage strokes using a massage cream to relax the first foot.
4. Apply gentle traction by holding the foot at the heel and pulling gently. Rotate the ankle clockwise and counterclockwise.
5. Using your thumb, work these key reflex points with firm but comfortable pressure:
   A. Big Toe Pad
   B. Ball of Foot
   C. Arch
   D. Heel
   E. Medial border
6. Make note of sensitive spots and cross reference them with the reflex chart. Give these spots more attention with the goal of rendering them less tender by the end of the session.
7. Finish with very- ight strokes wrap foot in a warm towel.

8. Repeat process on the other foot.
9. Have patient drink lots of water following the session.

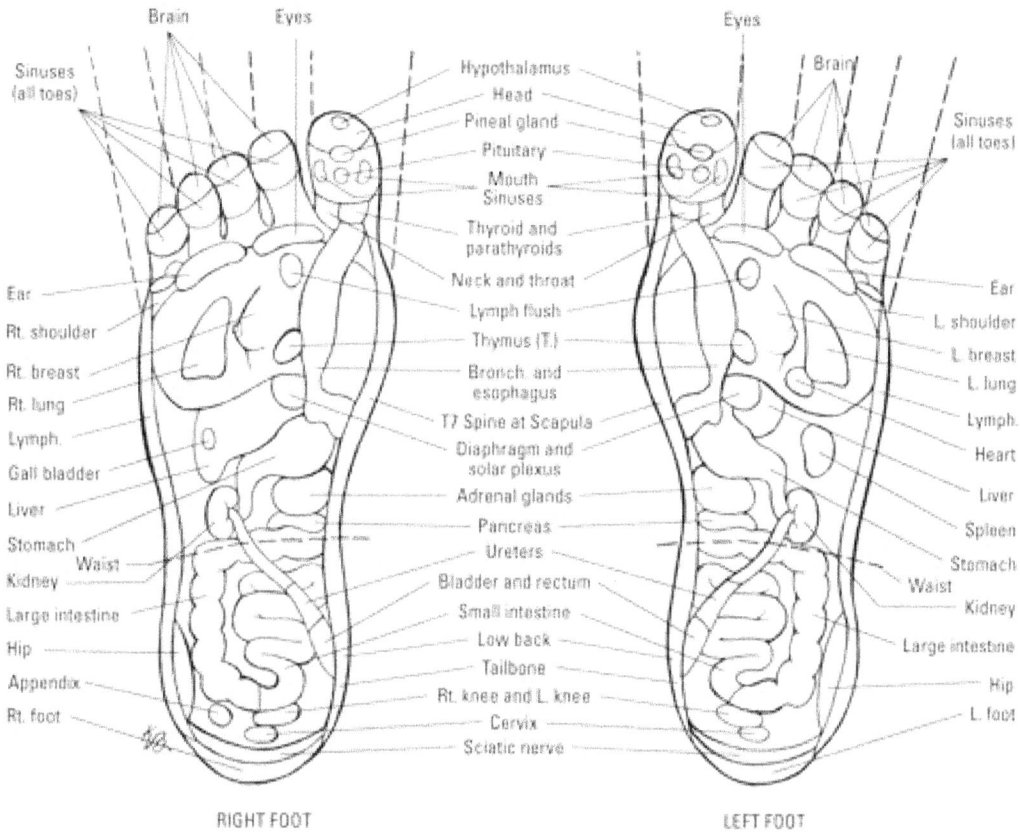

Brain   Eyes   Eyes   Brain

Sinuses (all toes)

Hypothalamus
Head
Pineal gland
Pituitary
Mouth
Sinuses
Thyroid and parathyroids
Neck and throat
Lymph flush
Thymus (T.)
Bronch. and esophagus
T7 Spine at Scapula
Diaphragm and solar plexus
Adrenal glands
Pancreas
Ureters
Bladder and rectum
Small intestine
Low back
Tailbone
Rt. knee and L. knee
Cervix
Sciatic nerve

Sinuses (all toes)

Ear
Rt. shoulder
Rt. breast
Rt. lung
Lymph.
Gall bladder
Liver
Stomach
Waist
Kidney
Large intestine
Hip
Appendix
Rt. foot

Ear
L. shoulder
L. breast
L. lung
Lymph.
Heart
Liver
Spleen
Stomach
Waist
Kidney
Large intestine
Hip
L. foot

RIGHT FOOT   LEFT FOOT

FREQUENCY OF TREATMENT
Dependent on the case, but not likely to over-treat.

REFERENCES
- Lucier, C. C., *Reflexology and Common Conditions: Methodology, Technique, Physiology, and Symptomatology*; 2025 The AtHome Experience
- Ingham, E., Byers, D.C., *Original Works of Eunice D. Ingham: Stories the Feet Can Tell Thru Reflexology/Stories the Feet Have Told Thru Reflexology*; 1984 Ingham Pub.
- Riley, J.S., *Zone Therapy Simplified*; 2010 Kessinger Pub. (Reprint)
- Lust, B., *Zone Therapy;* 1928 Benedict Lust Publications

MECHANOTHERAPY

SPONDYLOTHERAPY

DESCRIPTION

Dorland's Medical Dictionary defines Spondylotherapy as "physical methods applied to the spinal region; spinal therapeutics".

M

More specifically, it is a method of activating spinal reflexes without manipulating the spinal segments in the typical way. Instead, percussion is applied to the spinous processes, mechanically or by hand, using a reflex hammer, a mechanical vibrator or percussor, or sometimes just the hand. The ulnar side of the hand proximal to the 5th MCP joint has been used effectively as a percussion tool.

A.C. Johnson, DC, ND stated concisely in *Principles and Practice of Drugless Therapeutics*:

> "If the continuity of the nerve is interrupted or the molecular arrangement is disturbed by a mechanical stimulus, conduction of an impulse is interrupted and the excitability of a nerve is either diminished or extinguished. In conclusion, one may say that concussion of a short duration augments the excitability of the nerves, but, when prolonged, the excitability is diminished or abolished."

Although his contemporary Dr. George Starr White may have been the first, Albert Abrams, M.D., officially developed and named Spondylotherapy as a way of eliciting spinal response with minimal intervention. Alva Amory

Gregory, N.D., and Joe Shelby Riley, N.D., both elaborated on this technic for the naturopathic field. All four made contributions in the first third of the 20th Century to this simple method of treating the spine.

EQUIPMENT NEEDED
- Simply the hands; or
- A regular reflex testing rubber hammer and a thin firm pad; or
- A mechanical vibrator, set to low frequency and used through a few layers of towel

EFFECTS AND PURPOSE
The amplitude of the percussive force and the length of time it is applied will vary according to whether the appropriate nerve needs to be stimulated or inhibited. This is a concept in common with acupuncture, in which one "tonifies" (stimulates) or "sedates" (inhibits) the points.

INDICATIONS FOR USE
- Pain, spinal or referred along a dermatome.
- Organic dysfunction, using the spinal segments neurologically associated with the organ
- Malpositioned vertebra

CONTRAINDICATIONS
- Susceptibility to fractures (osteoporosis, bone infections, neoplasm, etc.)
- Bleeding disorders, or patients taking high doses of anticoagulant drugs.

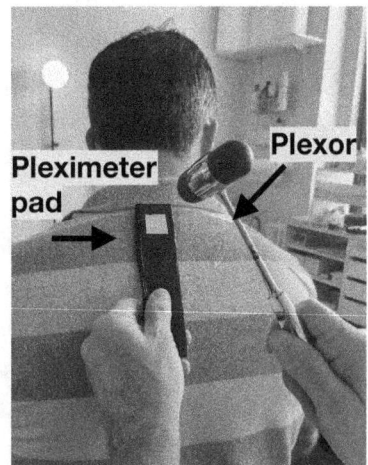

PRECAUTIONS
Ensure that the target is padded enough to receive the percussive impact, no matter how mild the strike. The pad is referred to as the *pleximeter* and the hammer as the *plexor*.

ADVANTAGES
- Spondylotherapy is a wonderful method for the traditional naturopath who may not have been trained in other spinal therapies such as manipulation. Particularly in those states where the Chiropractic lobby is strong and the

ND may find manipulation outside the scope of practice, this simple procedure allows you to use the spine as a treatment pathway without encroaching on other licenses.

- Two fingers can be used as the pleximeter and the clenched fist as the plexor, without resorting to any other equipment; therefore, ti can be applied anywhere.

DISADVANTAGES

The procedure will generally be unknown to the patient and an explanation is in order before proceeding. The patient will invariably compare it to Chiropractic and the distinction should be made clear.

INSTRUCTIONS

1. Explain that the purpose is not to move or re-position bones, but to excite spinal reflexes, which then do the work through the nervous system.
2. If it is a local problem, determine the exact spinal segment and record it.
3. Determine if stimulation or inhibition is to be used (local tenderness almost always calls for inhibition).
4. If it is organic dysfunction, refer to the following **Dermatome Map** to trace the problem area to a particular spinal segment, then consult the **Spinal Reflex Guide** to see on which spot to perform the Spondylotherapy percussion. The affiliated spinal segment or spinous process will typically be tender.
5. Extremely tender points can be treated with a steady pressure, gradually increasing the poundage of the pressure to the patient's tolerance. Steady pressure is especially indicated in spasm. Irritated areas may also be treated with cold applications; ice rubs, or spraying with refrigerants such as fluoromethane or ethyl chloride, are effective for quick relief of pain (Gebauer's **Spray and Stretch®** recommended).
6. To <u>stimulate</u> a spinal reflex and increase the activity of the nerves (in cases of hypofunction and numbness, paralysis, etc.), a short duration tapping is applied; up to 10 or so strokes. Tapping is applied two strokes per second for the duration, then paused for 30 seconds or so to allow for the response of the nerve reflex, then repeated three or four times.

7. To <u>inhibit</u> the spinal reflex (in the case of hyperactivity or pain), a longer duration is used; but still no more than 25-30 strokes. Tapping is once again applied more rapidly (four strokes per second for the duration, then paused for 30 seconds or so to allow for the response of the nerve reflex, then repeated. In inhibition, sometimes a third course of percussion is given.   Note: It is less tiring but no less effective to apply steady pressure to the spinal segment for several minutes instead of percussion or vibration.

8. In either stimulation or inhibition, the amplitude should be no more than 2-3 ounces of pressure.

- Inhibition may also be achieved by applying a **vapocoolant spray**, as mentioned above, to the spinal segment from 6-8 inches away, and held until the skin becomes white.
- Stimulation or inhibition may also be achieved by the use of the **High Frequency Plasma** device ("Violet Ray"). A spinal electrode is used that places two plasma tubes on opposing sides of a vertebra just over the nerve exit sites to activate visceral reflexes. Stimulation is achieved in 20-60 seconds (including sparking by lifting the bulb from the skin), and inhibition is achieved with 2-5 minutes duration.
- **Chromotherapy** can be applied to the spinal segment also to create spondylotherapy effects. Using a mask to narrow the light beam to just the vertebra in question, red light is applied in an intermittent manner for five minutes ti stimulate. To inhibit, blue light is applied in the same manner for an extended period of time; at least 30 minutes.
- **Vacuum Therapy** can also be applied to the nerve centers, over the chosen spinal segment for a short duration to stimulate, and for a longer duration (producing erythema) to inhibit.

One can see that many of the therapies covered in this book can be used for spondylotherapy.

FREQUENCY OF TREATMENT
Treatment can be applied daily if needed, until substantially improved

REFERENCES
- Colson, T., *Spondylotherapy Centers*, Electronic Medical Digest, 3rd quarter1953
- Johnson, A.C., *Principles and Practice of Drugless Therapeutics*; 3rd Ed., 1946 Chiropractic Educational Extension Bureau
- Abrams, A., *Spondylotherapy*, 1918 Philopolis Press
- Brown, B.H., *Vibratory Technique*, 2nd Edition, 1914 Vibratory Pub. Co., Chicago
- Snow, A., *Mechanical Vibration And Its Therapeutic Application*, 1904 Scientific Authors' Pub. Co.

DERMATOME MAP for SPONDYLOTHERAPY

ANTERIOR

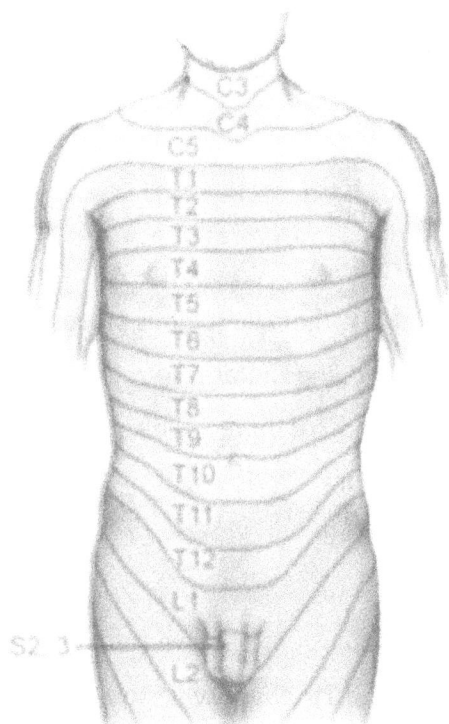

POSTERIOR

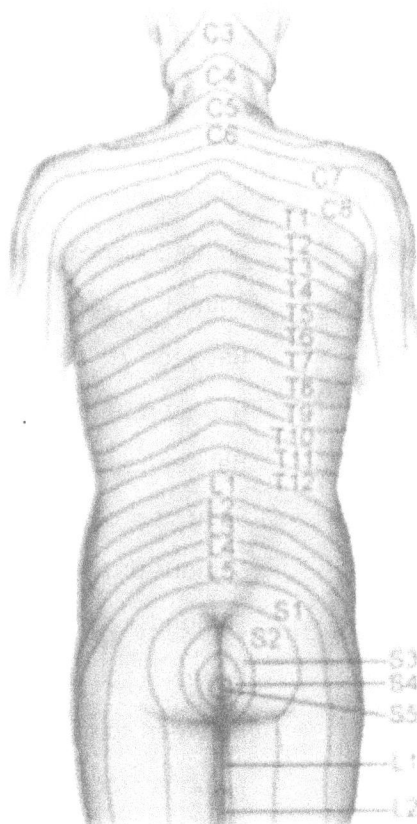

SPINAL REFLEX GUIDE

C1	Between occiput and spinous process of axis
C2	Middle of spinous process of axis
C3	End of spinous process of axis
C4	Spinous process of 3rd cervical vertebra
C5	Spinous process of 4th cervical vertebra
C6	Spinous process of 5th cervical vertebra
C7	Spinous process of 6th cervical vertebra
C8	Spinous process of 7th cervical vertebra
T1	Between 7th cervical vertebra and first thoracic spinous process
T2	Between spinous processes of 1st and 2nd thoracic vertebrae
T3	Between spinous processes of 2nd and 3rd thoracic vertebrae
T4	Spinous process of 3rd thoracic vertebra
T5	Spinous process of 4th thoracic vertebra
T6	Spinous process of 5th thoracic vertebra
T7	Between spinous processes of 5th and 6th thoracic vertebrae
T8	Between spinous processes of 6th and 7th thoracic vertebrae
T9	Spinous process of 7th thoracic vertebra
T10	Spinous process of 8th thoracic vertebra
T11	Between spinous processes of 9th and 10th thoracic vertebrae
T12	Spinous process of 11th thoracic vertebra
L1	Spinous process of 12th thoracic vertebra
L2	Between spinous processes of 1st and 2nd lumbar vertebrae
L3	Spinous process of 3rd lumbar vertebra
L4	Spinous process of 4th lumbar vertebra
L5	Spinous process of 5th lumbar vertebra

MECHANOTHERAPY

CHAPMAN'S REFLEXES

DESCRIPTION

Chapman's reflexes were discovered by Frank Chapman, DO. During his osteopathic practice in the early 20th Century, he noticed areas in the soft tissue that had a palpably different texture. He gradually realized that these were neurolymphatic reflex areas, and that they corresponded to specific viscera. Chapman was also able to make a correlation between these points and endocrinological functions. Chapman's reflexes are a similar phenomenon to what would come to be called trigger points, and are also what have been called *ah shi* points in acupuncture for centuries: tender spots that spontaneously appear when underlying tissues or organs are dysfunctional. The tenderness in the lymphoid tissue within the fascia is due to hypercongestion.

These viscerosomatic reflex points can be used to find an organic cause for a weak muscle found under examination / challenge. The neuromuscular connections to lymphoid tissue in the fascia have been mapped out.

EQUIPMENT NEEDED

Only hands.

EFFECTS AND PURPOSE

Chapman's reflexes are between the anterior and posterior fascia at specific points on the body, in the intercostal spaces. They feel tense when palpated. They are typically the size of a small bean, and are tender. For this last reason, they are diagnostic. They can be used for differential diagnosis of organic disease, as well as to regulate neurolymphatic communication to the affected organ.

INDICATIONS FOR USE
Any dysfunction.

CONTRAINDICATIONS
- Local trauma
- Bleeding tendency
-

PRECAUTIONS
Firm pressure and motion is used, but not hard enough to traumatize the tissues. The perceived power of the pressure by the subject is greater than the pressure perceived by the operator.

ADVANTAGES
- Gives the naturopath with a minimum of tools the ability to have a quick impact on symptoms
- Can be used for conditions ranging from adrenal or thyroid dysfunction to constipation—many of the common organic problems patients turn elsewhere for treatment
- Can be used anywhere for use outside the clinic, without equipment

DISADVANTAGES
None.

INSTRUCTIONS
1. Select points according to dysfunction; or...
2. Compare any tenderness found with the reflex chart to find the likely organic source.
3. Feel for a small
4. Make firm but gentle contact with the area to be treated with the pad of the finger.
5. Make gentle rotary motions while maintaining even pressure to "milk" the tissues of fluid and express it into the surrounding tissues. This reduces swelling, relieves the tenderness, and re-establishes a neurological "signal" to the affected viscera.

FREQUENCY OF TREATMENT

Can be repeated several times a day, depending on acuteness of symptoms.

REFERENCES

- Kuchera & Kuchera, *Osteopathic Considerations in Systemic Dysfunction*;. Greyden Press 1994
- Owen, Charles, *An Endocrine Interpretation of Chapman's Reflexes*; 1963 American Academy of Osteopathy

CHAPMAN'S REFLEXES CHARTS
(With kind permission of Pat Block, ND)

Unlike other segmented illustrations of Chapman's reflexes, this comprehensive chart is correlated with conditions and organs, which the practitioner can use to quickly arrive at the reflex points to use in a given case.

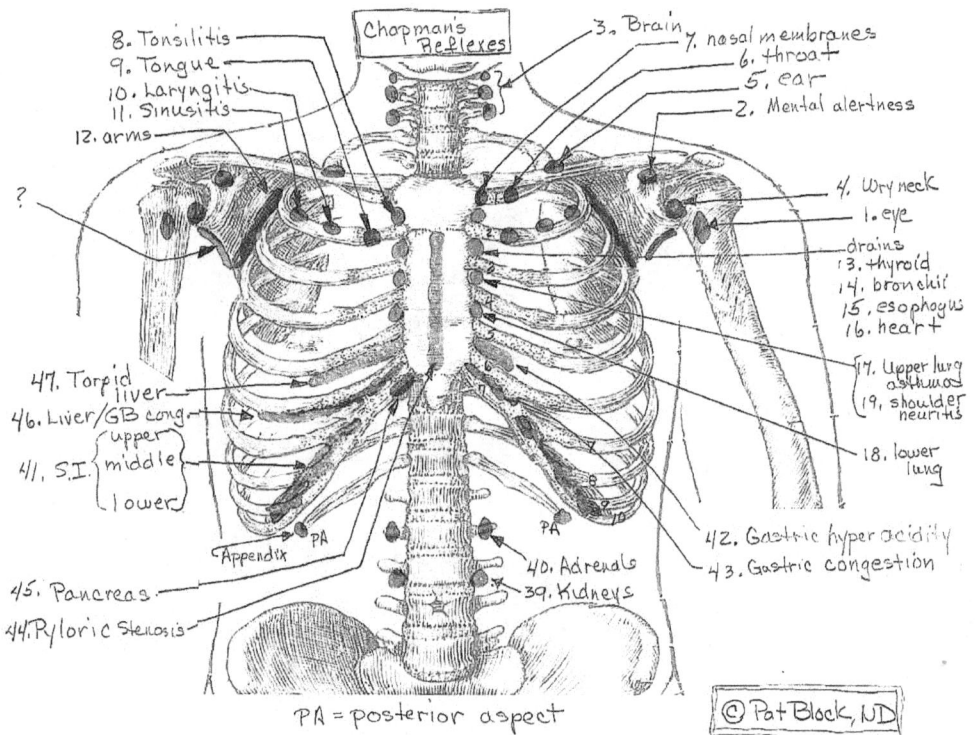

PA = posterior aspect

© Pat Block, ND

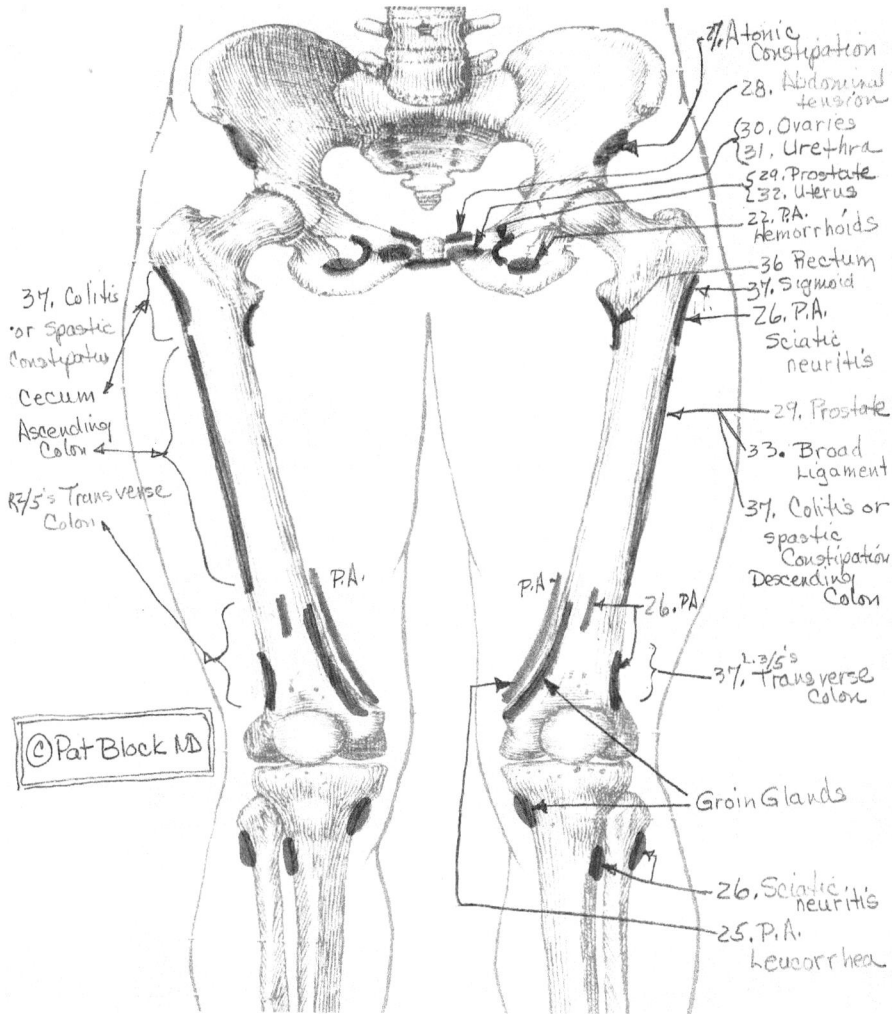

27. Atonic Constipation

28. Abdominal tension

30. Ovaries
31. Urethra
29. Prostate
32. Uterus

22. P.A. Hemorrhoids

36 Rectum
34. Sigmoid
26. P.A. Sciatic neuritis

29. Prostate

33. Broad Ligament

34. Colitis or spastic Constipation Descending Colon

34. Colitis or Spastic Constipation Cecum Ascending Colon

R3/5's Transverse Colon

P.A.

P.A.

26. P.A.

1.3/5's
34. Transverse Colon

© Pat Block MD

Groin Glands

26. Sciatic neuritis

25. P.A. Leucorrhea

MECHANOTHERAPY

NATUROPATHIC "BLOODLESS SURGERY"

DESCRIPTION

The best definition by G.E. Poesnecker, ND in *It's Only Natural*:
"A treatment that changes or alters the position or placement of
bodily parts without actually cutting the skin itself. "

M

Today, this is better known as "Deep Soft Tissue Manipulation". Most of the
time it is performed on the abdomen, however, Bloodless Surgery procedures
were originated by orthopedic surgeon Adolph Lorenz, MD to correct
deformities. He became famous in Germany, came to the USA to teach his
methods, and the technic passed on to naturopathic doctors like Joe Shelby
Riley, ND, Carl Frischkorn, ND, Harry Riley Spitler, ND, and Paul Wendel, ND
(who went on to write a
textbook devoted to it).

Lorenz made some of the
most remarkable
documented cures using
only his fingers, as
illustrated in the
photographs at right of a
child with congenital
deformities.

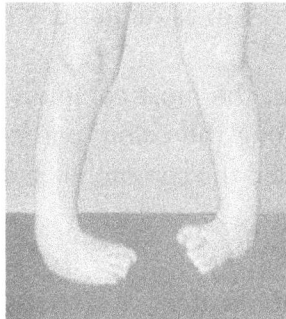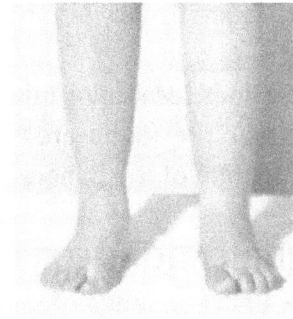

Before   After

By exerting the correct force on the connective tissue, he was able to break up adhesions and soften and lengthen tissues that allowed the normal tone to resume.

EQUIPMENT NEEDED
Hands alone.

EFFECTS AND PURPOSE
Adhesions for as a result of inflammation, or as a result of injury, or as a byproduct of surgery. When blood is forced to escape from its normal enclosure in the vessels, the clotting mechanism ensues. This is a natural self-protection instinct on the part of the body, for without we would bleed to death from an injury. The serum does not contain blood cells; however, it behaves very much like the clotting of blood. When forced into a space, it changes into a hardened consistency, much like an egg white is changed into a solid from a liquid. This plastic, sticky material hardens and begins to shrink. This formation is an adhesion. Bloodless Surgery uses a mechanical manipulation to break these adhesions and allow the tissues so adhered to each other to regain their normal positioning, whether muscular tissue or organic. It is virtually painless, as there is no innervation of the tissues in question.

Most of what you encounter is elastic tissue. True adhesions are partly fibrous tissue and are difficult to break, but elastic tissue can be severed with the fingers quite easily. Nevertheless, because they adhere to other tissues, they are usually also referred to as "adhesions".

Besides local joint injuries, the most common locations adhesions or elastic tissue are found are: Along the colon, particularly the splenic flexure; the junction of the pancreas and the common bile duct; and the Fallopian tubes.

INDICATIONS FOR USE
• Reduced range of joint motion
• Constipation
• Colitis
• Pyloric spasm
• Goiter
• Fibrositis

- Diverticulitis and diverticulosis
- Sluggish bile flow
- Entrapped gas
- Prostatic hyperplasia
- Prostate problems following prostatitis
- Prolapsed organs

CONTRAINDICATIONS
- Do not treat sites with a strong pain reaction.
- Do not treat over an area that presents a strong pulse beat.
- Do not treat over tumors.
- Do not treat patients with impaired sensation.
- Do not treat patient with a bleeding disorder.

PRECAUTIONS
See Contraindications.

ADVANTAGES
- Nothing needed but fingers
- Possible to effect dramatic changes in a short time

DISADVANTAGES
- Development of palpatory skills is necessary.

INSTRUCTIONS
The detection of adhesions by palpating its the fingers requires a decent length of time practicing. But, when the adhesions are pronounced, they can easily be felt by even a beginning operator. When palpating the abdomen, have the patient lie supine with the knees elevated.

1. Explain process to patient.
2. The <u>balls</u> of the fingers (not the tips) are used.
3. Palpate the problem area for nodules.
4. Determine if there is a lack of normal mobility of the parts being observed. When examining a joint, pay attention to the condition of the overlying soft tissues and not just the range of motion. The tissues may feel normal and smooth until you reach a specific site. Then you will feel a band or rope-like texture in the fascia.

Sometimes it presents as a series of knots. After trauma and strains, the fascia in the region sometimes maintains a buckled shape, and without a mechanical correction, remains as an adhesion.

5. Use your knowledge of anatomy to visualize the attachment soft the adhesions and which force(s) need to be applied in order to stretch and hopefully free them.

6. The five fingers of your non-dominant hand are placed flat at the site, and you give a deep pressure (equally distributed across all fingers) on the order of 10-15 pounds. You can test this on a bathroom scale until you get the "feel". The purpose of this pressure is to immobilize the offending tissue.   Anchor the target tissues with the balls of the fingers, holding them firmly. Sometimes it takes as much as 20-25 pounds pressure to stabilize the target.

7. The other hand is employed as the "scalpel". It is usually more efficient to use a pulling action toward you rather than pushing away. The fleshy part of the thumb is placed in contact with the index finger of the immobilizing hand, and pressed downward. Next, slide the thumb back and forth, using the edge of the index finger as the guide. Maintain the downward pressure throughout. You may feel a tearing or sudden relaxation of the connective tissue as a fibrous band snaps, and there may be an audible snapping sound.

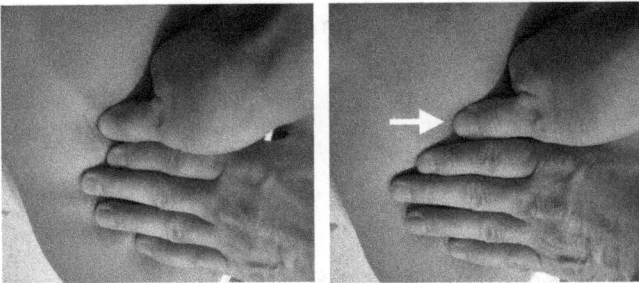

8.Patient should rest for (ideally) 30 minutes following procedure.

Generally, such elastic tissue being torn does not cause pain. The thing to remember is that this technic is contraindicated if there is severe pain experienced from simply palpating the site. If that is the case, lightly palpate and feel if there is a pulsation under the surface. If so, the local congestion must be reduced by other means so as not to cause internal hemorrhage by this maneuver.

The effect of this treatment continues to build over a week's time. It may take several sessions to achieve the results desired.

FREQUENCY OF TREATMENT
Once weekly until normalized.

REFERENCES
- Garten, M. O., *Health Secrets of a Naturopathic Doctor*; 1967 Parker Pub. Co.
- Lake, T. T., *Treatment By Neuropathy and The Encyclopedia of Manipulative Therapeutics*; 1946
- Wendel, P., *Naturopathic Bloodless Surgery with Technique and Treatments*; 1945 Wendel
- Lorenz, A., *My Life and Work*; 1936 Scribners

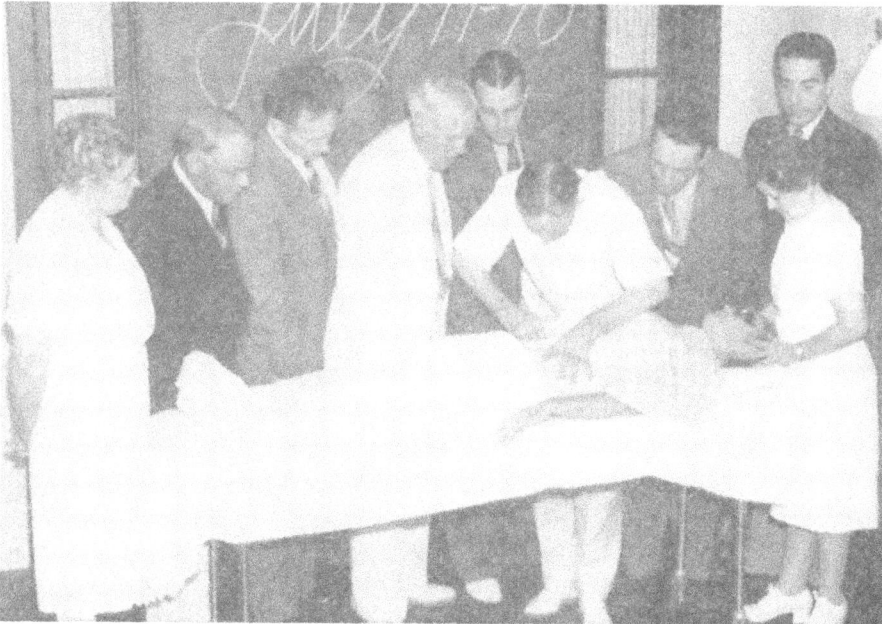

James McGinnis, ND, demonstrating Bloodless Surgery technic.

MECHANOTHERAPY

PNEUMATIC (VACUUM) THERAPY

DESCRIPTION

Today, Pneumatic or Vacuum Therapy is associated with Asian medical practices (and called "Cupping"), and while it has historically been used in those disciplines for hundreds of years, naturopaths were using this as a scientifically sound physiotherapy from the 1920s through the 1940s—long before anyone in the U.S. had heard of acupuncture.

M

Essentially, the operator places glass or plastic bells on the patient's back, stomach, arms, legs or other regions. A vacuum or suction force inside the cup pulls the skin upward inside the bell or cup. Blood is drawn up to the surface of the skin and away from congested tissues, moving along metabolic waste, removing obstacles to lymph flow, and generally fulfilling the naturopathic principles of therapy: removing toxins and regulating the natural processes of the body.

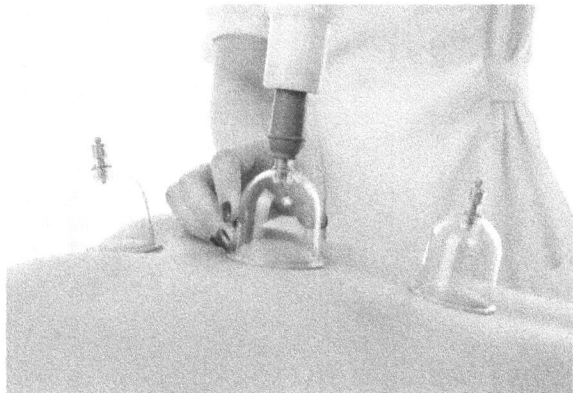

It should be noted that in current surgical practice, deep wounds are being sealed using vacuum therapy (sometimes called "negative pressure wound therapy" or "vacuum assisted closure") that is indistinguishable from our natural methodology.

EQUIPMENT NEEDED

- A set of different size bells ("cups") for various applications, and a vacuum device made for drawing the air out through a connecting hose (some simpler sets use a hand-operated pump)
- Materials for sterilizing the contact points between usages

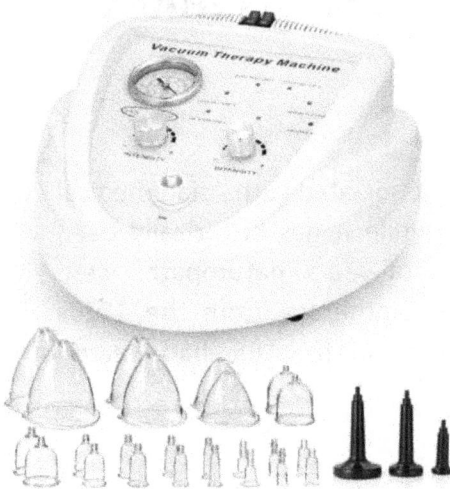

EFFECTS AND PURPOSE

•Breaks up congestion of blood beneath the site
•Stimulates the peripheral nervous system
•Increases erythrocyte formation
•Aids detoxification

INDICATIONS FOR USE

- Fatigue
- Muscle weakness
- Back, neck, and limb pain
- Headaches
- Reduce inflammation
- Relax tight muscles
- Increase range of motion of joints
- Improve local peripheral circulation
- Create visceral reflex actions

CONTRAINDICATIONS

- Patients with bleeding tendency or on blood-thinning drugs
- Patients with polycythemia vera
- Skin infections
- Skin conditions like eczema or psoriasis
- History of stroke or cardiovascular disease
- Epilepsy

PRECAUTIONS

The form of cupping that uses a flame to evacuate the air in the cups is archaic and dangerous and is not recommended.

CUPPING SITES

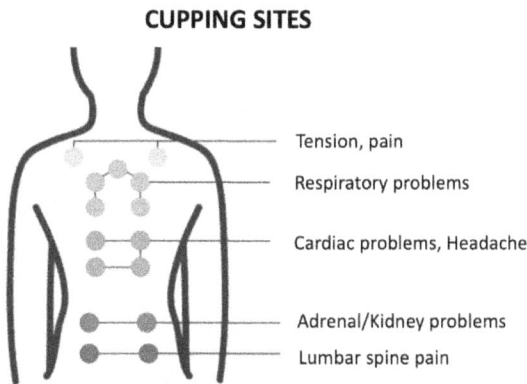

Tension, pain
Respiratory problems
Cardiac problems, Headache
Adrenal/Kidney problems
Lumbar spine pain

ADVANTAGES
• "Low tech"
• Minimal skill required

DISADVANTAGES
• Can cause unsightly bruising
• Associated by the medical profession with pseudo-scientific practices

INSTRUCTIONS

1. Choose appropriate site according to the complaint or visceral neurotome (Vacuum Therapy may be applied to the side of spinal segments as detailed in **Spondyotherapy**).
2. Disinfect the skin at the site, checking for any abnormality that would contraindicate Vacuum therapy.
3. Choose a suitable size bell for the site.
4. Apply bell and connect the hose or hand-held vacuum gun.
5. Draw out the air and seal the opening. Disconnect pump and repeat at each site needed.
6. Leave bells/cups on for 10-15 minutes.
7. Remove cups by releasing the piston seals.
8. Wipe cups with disinfectant.

FREQUENCY OF TREATMENT

Once weekly

REFERENCES

• Johnson, A.C., *Principles and Practice of Drugless Therapeutics*; 3rd Ed., 1946 Chiropractic Educational Extension Bureau
• Lake, T. T., *Treatment By Neuropathy and The Encyclopedia of Manipulative Therapeutics*; 1946

MECHANOTHERAPY

MANUAL TRACTION

DESCRIPTION

Spinal traction is commonly used in orthopedic medicine, Chiropractic and Physical Therapy, but the motorized form is typically employed. There are two types: *intersegmental traction* (such as the famous Spinalator table), which lifts and stretches individual spinal segments to reduce fixations, and *long axis motorized traction*, which is a more profound and efficacious method of reducing neurological deficits from discogenic conditions.

Long axis traction can also be done manually, and it was this form that has been more associated with naturopathic doctors. The technic, like motorized traction, creates space between the vertebrae, enhancing blood flow and relieving the discomfort caused by spinal compression. The practitioner uses the hands, sometimes aided by straps, to create the traction. In the case of the cervical spine, a towel is often used as the strap.

A distinction between the way the naturopath uses traction and other practitioners is that the naturopathic form is intermittent. Static traction, as applied in hospitals and physical therapy clinics, maintains a pull at a specific poundage for 20 minutes or so. Naturopathic manual traction uses a gentle oscillation to open and decompress the spinal segments, for short durations. It should take about four seconds to make one complete oscillation and return to the start point; put another way, 12 complete maneuvers per minute.

The poundage of pull is a critical critical matter in static and motorized traction. The traditional rule is 5% of the patient's body weight for cervical traction, 25% for lumbar traction. While this may or may not be adhered to in practice, the starting poundage for cervical traction on an adult is usually 15 pounds and 50 pounds for lumbar. Obviously, less weight is used depending on age, size, weight, and sex. It is generally agreed that the maximum poundage for the cervical spine is 60 pounds (for a large male patient) and 125 pounds for lumbar.

In manual traction, poundage is a subjective matter for both the operator and the patient. Therefore, the procedure is to:

- Secure a good hold
- Check that the proper angle is adopted, according to the target area (see **instructions**, below)
- Ask patient to signal when a strong stretch is felt (or relief, and certainly if pain occurs—in which case, discontinue)
- Begin the pull slowly and gradually without wavering
- When patient signals, hold for a second, then pull slightly stronger for two seconds, and return to original degree of pull for another two seconds.
- Without going lower than the original poundage, repeat the oscillations (two seconds increase, two seconds return) for 1-7 minutes

It is important to mention that cases with radiculitis from either cervical or lumbar impairment should be treated with electrical stimulation following the traction. This will decrease any muscular reaction to the traction and passively exercise the affected muscles. This will treat the soft tissue associated with the affected segment(s) without putting the joints themselves through further range of motion. It will rehabilitate the soft tissues while calming the affected nerve roots. A surging Faradic or sine wave current are the best choices (see **electrotherapy**).

EQUIPMENT NEEDED
- Hands
- Towel
- Straps of strong woven material, in a variety of widths and lengths

EFFECTS AND PURPOSE
- Stretching of the paraspinal ligaments and muscles
- Increasing the tension of the longitudinal ligament, leading to restore the elastic response of the outer portion of the disk (*annulus fibrosis*)
- Distraction of the vertebral bodies to enlarge the intervertebral space and create a suction effect to draw disk tissue into its proper position
- Pumping and hydrating the disks

INDICATIONS FOR USE
- Acute intervertebral disk-related pain
- Chronic degenerative joint disease
- Hip osteoarthritis
- Sciatica
- Myospasm

CONTRAINDICATIONS
- Pregnancy
- Spinal cord compression
- Infectious disease of the spine
- Active peptic ulcers
- Aortic aneurysm
- Hernia
- Spinal osteoporosis
- Metastatic malignancy

PRECAUTIONS
- Obviously, the wrong poundage of pull is counter-productive, but the wrong angle of pull is more often the cause of discomfort or poor results.
- Before beginning traction therapy, the patient should have been treated for any gross vertebral misalignment or rotation
- Severe myospasm should be treated with static action rather than intermittent manual traction, as the oscillations could worsen the spasm.

ADVANTAGES
- Manual traction can produce dramatic results with difficult cases that only marginally respond to other mechanotherapy procedures.
- Can be done manually with or without strap.

DISADVANTAGES
Requires a certain degree of strength and endurance, but use of straps makes the technic more efficient to the extent that even a naturopath of slight build can effectively deliver benefit without exhaustion.

INSTRUCTIONS

Cervical traction:

1. Place bolster under knees of supine patient.
2. Ideally, strap patient's hips to the table.
3. Obtain hold with either hands, towel or strap.
4. Precisely raise the head to the degree of angle indicated by the spinal segment(s) restricted (see next page).
5. Ask patient to signal when a strong stretch is felt (or relief, and certainly if pain occurs—in which case, discontinue)
6. Begin the pull slowly and gradually without wavering
7. When patient signals, hold for a second, then pull slightly stronger for two seconds, and return to original degree of pull for another two seconds.
8. Without going lower than the original poundage, repeat the oscillations (two seconds increase, two seconds return) for 1-7 minutes

ANGULATION—CERVICAL

#1 illustrates how a cervical spine with hypolordosis can be benefitted with traction. The spine is held in slight extension at negative angulation. Note the chin is raised.

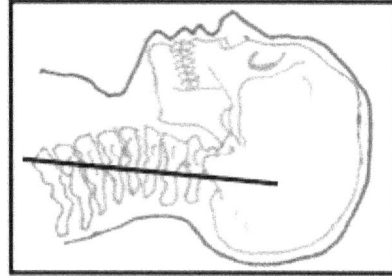

①
-5° to
-10°

#2 shows how the spine with zero angulation targets the occiput and upper cervicals.

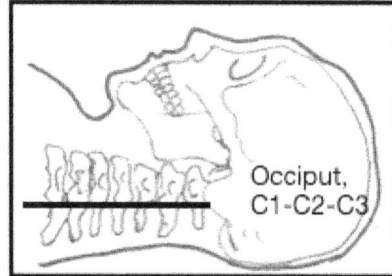

②
0°

Occiput,
C1-C2-C3

#3 flexes the spine five to fifteen degrees, taking the pull off the occiput and opening the top three vertebrae.

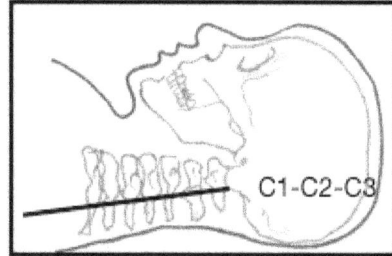

③
5° to
15°

C1-C2-C3

#4 increases the flexion further and one can see from the illustration how this distracts C4, C5, and C6.

Notice that the more the chin is tucked, the lower the vertebrae that are distracted.

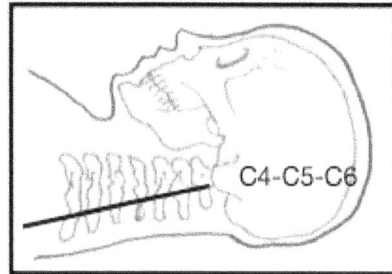

④
30°

C4-C5-C6

#5 at a 50 degree angulation, not only are the three lower cervical vertebrae distracted, but also the top three thoracic vertebrae as well: T1, T2, and T3.

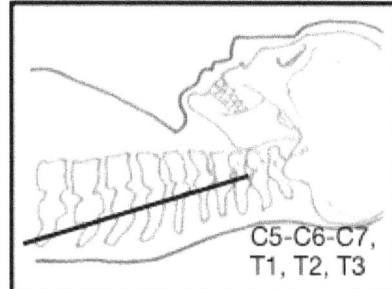

⑤
50°

C5-C6-C7,
T1, T2, T3

Lumbar traction:
1. Place bolster under knees of supine patient.
2. Secure strap across patient's waist to hold hips to the table
3. Ideally also strap the patient to the table at chest level
4. Obtain hold with either hands, towel or strap.
5. Precisely raise the legs to the degree of angle indicated by the spinal segment(s) restricted (see next page).
6. Ask patient to signal when a strong stretch is felt (or relief, and certainly if pain occurs—in which case, discontinue)
7. Begin the pull slowly and gradually without wavering
8. When patient signals, hold for a second, then pull slightly stronger for two seconds, and return to original degree of pull for another two seconds.
9. Without going lower than the original poundage, repeat the oscillations (two seconds increase, two seconds return) for 1-7 minutes

ANGULATION—LUMBAR

#1 illustrates how an oblique raising of the legs at 15 degrees isolates and distracts the lower thoracic vertebrae and the upper two lumbars

#2 shows how training the legs to 30 degrees begins to reduce the lumbar lordosis and separate L2, L3, and L4.

#3 position, with the legs raised the highest at 50 degrees, now flattens the lumbar curve and distracts L3, L4, L5, and S1.

1
15°

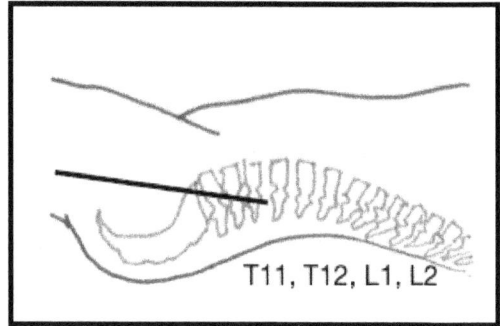

T11, T12, L1, L2

2
30°

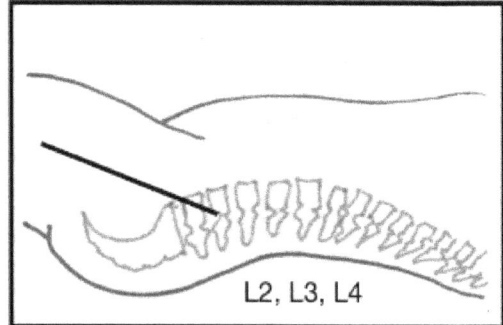

L2, L3, L4

3
50°

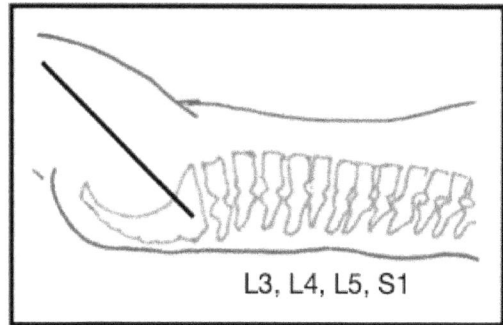

L3, L4, L5, S1

FREQUENCY OF TREATMENT

For the fastest response in acute cases, it is recommended to treat three consecutive days, and then 2-3 sessions a week for 6-8 weeks. Chronic cases may need 1-2 sessions weekly for a more protracted length of time. 10-20 treatments is typical.

REFERENCES

- McElhannon, J., *A Guide to Physio-therapeutics*; 1984 McElhannon
- DeStephano, L., Greenman's *Principles of Manual Medicine*; 4th Ed., 2011 Walters Kluwer

9

Clinical Decision Making

With the array of modalities at the disposal of the naturopathic doctor, one will naturally develop favorites. However, a solid study of these methods will often show a distinct advantage of one over the other in a particular case. Certain maladies respond better to one kind of treatment than another and this is well documented in the allopathic literature as well as the naturopathic literature. All types of clinicians tend to attract the cases that they do best with; a familiarity with more modalities means a greater scope of practice and a broader potential service to the public.

The following chart is a quick guide to the best therapy to apply for the condition at hand.

Physiotherapy Modalities and Their Use in Musculoskeletal Complaints

Therapy	Contusion	Strain	Sprain	Spasm	Tendonitis	Bursitis	Arthritis	Neuralgia	Fibromyalgia
Rest	●	●	●	●	●	●	●	●	●
Acupuncture	●	●	●	●	●	●	●	●	●
Cold Hydro	1	1	1					●	
Hot Hydro	2	●	2	●	●		●		●
Infrared	2	●	2	●	●	●	●	●	●
Ultraviolet	●		●		●	●	●	●	●
Electric light						●	●		●
Artif. sunlight	●		●		●	●	●	●	●
Sunlight	●	●	●	●	●	●	●	●	●
Laser	●	●	●		●	●	●	●	●
Chromotherapy	●	●	●	●	●	●	●	●	●
Massage	2	●	2	●	●	2	2		●
Manipulation				●				●	●
Vibrotherapy	●	●	2	●	●	2	2	●	●
Galvanic	-	+	+	●	+		●	+	●
Sine				●					
High Freq	●	●	●		●	●	●	●	●
Diathermy	2	●	2	●	●	●	●	●	●
Ultrasound	2	●	2	●	●	●	●	●	●

1=First stage treatment 2 = Second stage treatment, after acute inflammation subsides
+ =Positive polarity current − = Negative polarity current ● = Indicate

www.ingramcontent.com/pod-product-compliance
Lightning Source LLC
Chambersburg PA
CBHW081432270326
41932CB00019B/3179